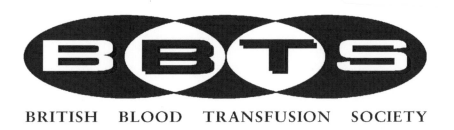

BRITISH BLOOD TRANSFUSION SOCIETY

AN INTRODUCTION TO

BLOOD TRANSFUSION SCIENCE

AND

BLOOD BANK PRACTICE

Phil Learoyd
Robin Knight
Peter Rogan
Martin Haines

Fifth Edition: March 2009

British Blood Transfusion Society
Enterprise House, Manchester Science Park,
Manchester M15 6SE

An Introduction to Blood Group Serology and Blood Bank Practice
First edition published in Great Britain in January 1996 by BBTS
Reprinted and Revised in January 1998 by BBTS

An Introduction to Blood Group Serology and Blood Bank Practice
Second (revised) edition published in Great Britain in January 2000 by BBTS

An Introduction to Blood Transfusion Science and Blood Bank Practice
Third (revised) edition published in Great Britain in January 2002 by BBTS

Fourth (revised) edition published in Great Britain in 2006 by BBTS
Reprinted in 2007

Fifth (revised) edition published in Great Britain in 2009 by BBTS

A CIP catalogue record for this book is available from the British Library.

ISBN 978 0 9512691 5 2

Printed in Great Britain by:

British Blood Transfusion Society (BBTS)
Enterprise House
Manchester Science Park
Lloyd Street North
Manchester
M15 6SE
www.bbts.org.uk

CONTENTS

INTRODUCTION

This edition represents a major re-writing of this book and (like the fourth edition) includes an update and increase in the information regarding blood donation testing and processing, as well as some additional specialist transfusion science information. This has been done in response to continuing changes and evolution of the BBTS examination from the 'Certificate' to the 'Specialist' scheme, which has resulted in extending the amount of material to encompass the needs of staff working for the Blood Services, as well as those in hospital based transfusion science. One obvious effect of these changes is the additional fourth author, Mr Martin Haines, who has contributed a revised specialist Blood Components section.

The British Blood Transfusion Society (BBTS) continues to be committed to supporting training and education. In response to changing educational requirements in the UK with regard to pathology sciences, the BBTS has revised its 'Certificate' course and examination into a Specialist Certificate in Transfusion Science Practice. As such, this training is aimed at UK Health Professions Council (HPC) registered scientists who are looking to specialise in Transfusion Science. The 'training package' reflects the training standards expressed as learning outcomes. The training guide details the topics that should be covered by the student, together with suggested guidelines as well as other references that should be read / consulted, since they contain what the authors consider to be essential information for anyone performing specialist laboratory transfusion science. Therefore, whilst the training standards define what needs to be achieved, the study guide helps you to plan, together with a senior member of your laboratory staff, your own learning programme.

This book is designed to provide basic Transfusion Science information related to the knowledge requirements identified in the Study Guide. It is envisaged that the student however will need to supplement the material contained within this book with information available from standard textbooks and/or the relevant published guidelines that are referenced in this book. The information provided within this book is intended for use in conjunction with in-service practical training.

QUESTIONS AND ANSWERS

At the end of each section of this book there are a number of questions for you to answer. To make the best use of this book, read each section in turn, answering the questions in writing before looking at the answers (which are at the back of the book). It is recommended that the guidelines and other references relevant to the section (identified within the text) are also read. If you have not understood something, it is recommended that you go back and read the section again and, if possible, read about the subject in one of the recommended textbooks, before moving onto the next section.

ASSIGNMENTS

At the end of some sections of this book there is a suggested assignment for which there are no answers given, but if possible, they should be discussed with your work place supervisor. The completion of these assignments will enable you to gain a better understanding of the subject but do not form part of any formal assessment.

Note:
You must make yourself aware of the policies and procedures used in your own laboratory. Please note however that these may differ in some respects to those given in this book. Guidelines, produced by the BBTS and the British Committee for the Standardisation in Haematology (BCSH), are listed in the 'Sources of Additional Information' section and these too should be read in conjunction with this book.

ACKNOWLEDGEMENTS

The authors are indebted to Ms Robina Qureshi (Liverpool Blood Centre) and Mr Mark Williams (Leeds Blood Centre) for their invaluable help in preparing this edition as well as to Mr Andy Miller (North London Blood Centre) for providing the illustrations.

If you have any problems, questions or comments about this book, please direct them to the authors via the BBTS, Enterprise House, Manchester Science Park, Manchester M15 6SE. Telephone number 0161 2327999.

SECTION 1

ANTIGEN - ANTIBODY REACTIONS

DEFINITIONS

ANTIGEN: Any substance, which in appropriate biological circumstances can stimulate an immune response, e.g. the formation of an antibody or the activation of antigen specific effector cells.

ANTIBODY: Proteins occurring in body fluids which are produced in response to the introduction of a foreign antigen.

An antigen - antibody reaction is specific, i.e. a given antibody specificity will react only with its corresponding antigen.

WHAT ARE BLOOD GROUP ANTIGENS?

Blood group antigens are located within many red cell membrane structures and are inherited characteristics. Inheritance of different genetic material results in the production of different blood group antigens, i.e. ABO, Rh, etc. The presence of alternative genes (alleles) at these genetic loci (produced as a result of genetic mutation) results in the production of alternative antigenic material, e.g. A or B antigens of the ABO blood group system. Red cell antigens are therefore variable (alternative) parts of the red cell membrane, the vast majority of which do not appear to affect red cell function.

       The blood group genes, via mRNA, either code for red cell membrane proteins directly (e.g. Rh antigens), or code for enzymes, which cause the production of specific red cell membrane carbohydrate sugars (e.g. A and B antigens).

RED CELL MEMBRANE COMPOSITION

The red cell membrane is composed of approximately equal amounts of lipid (~44%) and protein (~49%), together with a small amount (~7%) of carbohydrate.

Lipid

The major (approximately 75%) lipid component of the red cell membrane is phospholipid, which are molecules having hydrophilic (water-soluble) polar ("head") groups and two hydrophobic (water insoluble) low viscosity chain ("tail") groups. The hydrophobic areas align to form a basic phospholipid bi-layer structure, which is approximately 7nm across. This structure provides the red cell membrane with its major properties of impermeability (i.e. to ions, water and metabolites) and fluidity (i.e. flexibility and deformability within the plane of the membrane).

Protein

The presence of protein within the phospholipid bi-layer provides the capacity for selective transport across the membrane barrier, as well as providing a skeletal function. The protein may be extrinsic (projecting above the phospholipid bi-layer) or intrinsic (on the inside or across the phospholipid bi-layer), or both. Red cell protein may be free within the phospholipid bi-layer or anchored to protein (e.g. ankrin and spectrin) lying underneath the phospholipid bi-layer.

Carbohydrate

The carbohydrate present in the red cell membrane is associated with either protein, (i.e. as glycoprotein), or with lipid (i.e. as glycolipid). The ABO, Lewis, P and H antigen structures are carbohydrate structure whereas the Rh, Kell, Duffy, Kidd and Lutheran antigens are glycoprotein structures.

Glycoprotein structures are mainly long chain structures (e.g. sialoglycoprotein) extending above the red cell membrane surface. These molecules contain most of the red cell membrane sialic acid (i.e. N-acetyl-neuraminic acid). Sialic acid is one of the major charged molecules of the red cell membrane. Glycoprotein comprises the major charged molecules within the red cell membrane and as such it confers the red cell with a net negative charge.

The most common types of red cell sialoglycoprotein are glycophorin A (GPA), which includes the MN antigen structures and glycophorin B (GPB), which includes the Ss antigen structures. Since these rod-like glycoprotein structures extend some distance above the red cell membrane, some of them are (like the Duffy glycoprotein) sensitive to proteolytic enzyme treatment (e.g. by papain).

Glycolipid molecules form only approximately 5% of the total lipid presence of the red cell membrane and are known as sphingosine molecules (i.e. long chain fatty acids).

Schematic cross-sectional representation of the red cell membrane structure to illustrate some of the membrane glycoproteins (not to scale)

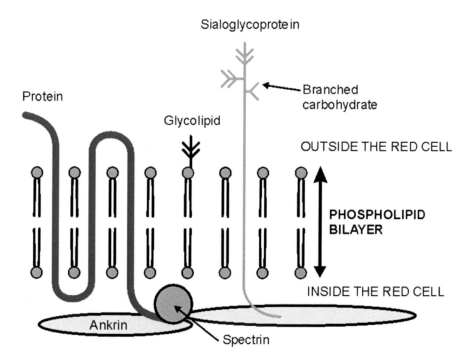

Blood group antigens can be identified to be present as alternative molecules within a variety of specific red cell membrane structures:

NAME	ASSOCIATED MEMBRANE STRUCTURE *	CHROMOSOME GENE LOCUS
ABO	Carbohydrate	9
MNS	Sialoglycoprotein (GPA / GPB)	4
P	Glycolipid	22
Rh	Proteins	1
Lutheran	Glycoprotein	19
Kell	Glycoprotein	7
Lewis	Carbohydrate	19
Duffy	Glycoprotein	1
Kidd	Glycoprotein	18

* For further information regarding the functions associated with these red cell membrane structures, refer to information on the individual blood group systems.
  GPA = Glycophorin A / GPB = Glycophorin B

INDIVIDUAL ANTIGEN SPECIFICITIES

The difference between antithetical blood group antigens has been identified in some instances to be due to very minor differences within the 'parent' protein. For example, the M and N antigen structure difference is produced by a change to two amino acids (at positions 1 and 5) within glycophorin A, a protein consisting of 131 amino acids. The difference between the S and s antigens is due to a single amino acid change at position 29 within glycophorin B, a protein consisting of 72 amino acids.

Representation of some of the major red cell membrane glycoproteins and variations in antigenic structures (not to scale)

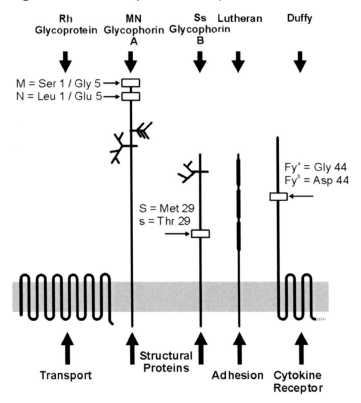

These differences do not appear to affect the specific function of the different 'parent' glycoprotein structures, e.g. in their structural, receptor molecule, trans-membrane transport function.

The very minor structural variations associated with some antithetical antigens, though capable of eliciting an antibody response in some patients is reflected in (to some degree) to their relatively low immunogenicity. This situation is in sharp contrast to the immunogenicity of the RhD protein, which has no antithetical antigen option (i.e. *D* has no allelic gene option). As such, the presence of the RhD protein of D+ red cells will be more immunogenic to a D- recipient, accounting for the high immunogenicity of the RhD protein, compared with other (non-ABO) red cell antigens.

Therefore 'red cell antigens' can be identified to be associated with specific red cell membrane structures, the majority of which have been shown to have a specific function, i.e.

RED CELL FUNCTION	BLOOD GROUPS
Membrane transport	Rh, Kidd, Kx, Diego, Colton
Membrane bound enzymes	Kell, Cartwright
Structural / assembly	MNSs, Gerbich
Chemokine receptor	Duffy
Cell adhesion molecules	Lutheran, LW, Xg, Indian
Complement regulation	Cromer, Knops

Notes: Colton: Membrane water transport protein (Aquaporin-1 or AQP/CHIP).
Lewis and Chido/Rodgers (as C4) are adsorbed onto red cells.
Dombrock: function unknown.

Since an antigenic specificity may be defined by something as small as a single carbohydrate (e.g. A and B antigens) or alternative amino-acids within a single protein (e.g. M and N antigens), each red cell expresses an enormous number of each antigen on its surface, i.e.

BLOOD GROUP	ANTIGEN	APPROXIMATE NUMBER OF ANTIGEN SITES PER RED CELL *
ABO	A	810,000 - 1,200,000
	B	600,000 – 850,000
Rh	D	10,000 - 40,000
Kell	K	3,000 - 4,000
Duffy	Fy^a	10,000 - 15,000

* Calculated by radioisotope (^{125}I) labelled antibody binding and flow cytometry experiments (performed by a number of different research groups).

Generally, the same antibody binding experiments have demonstrated that more antigen sites are detectable on red cells of the homozygote rather than the heterozygote phenotype, i.e.

DD homozygote: approximately 25,000 - 37,000 sites per red cell.
Dd heterozygote: approximately 10,000 - 15,000 sites per red cell.

This factor is a major reason why homozygous antigen expression is preferred for the red cells that are used for antibody detection, since they offer a potential for improved reactivity.

The location and number of antigen sites on each red cell can affect antigen-antibody reactivity in a variety of ways:

a. The type of laboratory technique able to be used to demonstrate the antigen-antibody reaction (i.e. IgG ABO antibodies reacting by saline techniques compared with anti-human globulin (AHG) and/or enzyme used for the detection of IgG Rh antibodies).

b. The effects of the action of enzymes (e.g. papain) on the antigen - antibody reaction, i.e. as to whether antigen-antibody reactivity is enhanced (e.g. Rh) or destroyed (e.g. Duffy).

c. The strength (avidity) of the antigen-antibody reaction produced, i.e. the ease with which the antibody is able to react with its antigen.

ANTIBODY PRODUCTION

Antibodies are immunoglobulins (proteins) which are produced when an antigenic structure is recognised by the immune system as foreign. This process involves a series of interrelated stages, which form the 'humoral' rather than 'cellular' part of the immune response mechanism. Basically, the antigen is processed by antigen presenting cells (APC), normally macrophages. The processed antigen (antigen fragment or epitope) is presented by the APC, together with a glycoprotein coded for by the Major Histocompatibility Complex (MHC), to a CD4+ (helper) T lymphocyte. These in turn inter-react with other cells, resulting in the activation of a B lymphocyte into growth and differentiation to become a plasma cell. It is the plasma cells that synthesise and secrete antibody molecules, which are specific for the antigen structure that stimulated their production. The amount and type / subtype of immunoglobulin produced results from the interaction of CD4+ (T-helper) and CD8+ (T-suppressor) lymphocytes. The antibody produced reacts with and is (normally) specific for the structure of the antigen that stimulated its production. This mechanism results in the production of a 'unique' antibody specificity (i.e. the "lock and key" theory).

A variable (large) number of B lymphocytes may be involved in each immune response, since many red cell antigens are complex structures containing different portions (epitopes), many of which are able to be recognised as immunogenic by the immune system. A number of plasma cells (clones) may therefore be stimulated to secrete antibody, which is aimed at a single antigenic specificity. As such, the immune response is said to be 'polyclonal', i.e. the production of a heterogeneous mixture of 'anti-epitope' antibody molecules with similar but not identical specificities. Invariably, this is however of little practical importance in the transfusion laboratory since these (anti-epitope polyclonal) antibodies are identified as a 'single antibody' against a single red cell antigen specificity.

The immune response in man, which results in the production of antibody, is highly individualistic. How well it works, or even if it works at all, is dependent upon a variety of factors, e.g. the amount and immunising capability ('immunogenicity') of the antigen, the immune responsiveness of the patient and a number of genetic effects, i.e. the presence of certain HLA-DR (class II) genes. The production of antibody, involving circulating monocytes, T and B lymphocytes and tissue bound macrophages, may result from either a primary and/or secondary response.

Primary response

This immune response is produced as a result of the first antigen encounter, and 'classically' results in the production, after a relatively lengthy delay (several weeks to several months), of small amounts of IgM antibody, with the production subsequently changing over to IgG antibody molecules. However, this is a generalisation with regard to the primary immune response to some red cell antigens (e.g. RhD), which may involve the relatively rapid production of mainly IgG antibody.

Once antibody has been produced, some B cells have the capability to act as long lived primed ('memory') cells, which remain in the circulation. Antigen processing of transfused red cells by splenic macrophages probably only occurs when the red cells are removed from the patient's circulation at the end of their normal life span, which adds to the delay prior to antibody production.

Summary of the primary immune response process

Immunisation by (foreign) antigen

↓

Contact of antigen with an Antigen Presenting Cell (APC)

↓

Antigen ingested, processed (broken down) and presented on the outer surface of the APC together with Major Histocompatibility Complex (MHC) class II protein

↓

Reaction of the APC with a CD4+ T-helper lymphocyte that recognises the foreign antigen in combination with the MHC receptor protein

↓

APC secretes interleukin-1 (IL-1) stimulating the CD4+ cell to secrete cytokines and interferon, which stimulate proliferation of more T lymphocytes - though this may be inhibited by activation of CD8+ T-suppressor lymphocytes

↓

Secretion of B cell growth factor and binding to the activated CD4+ cell stimulates a B lymphocyte to divide and produce genetically identical daughter cells

↓

Daughter cells develop into plasma (antibody secreting) cells and memory cells

APCs secrete interleukin-1 (IL-1), which stimulates CD4+ cells to enlarge and begin to secrete cytokines allowing proliferation and stimulation of more T cells. Secreted B cell growth factor stimulates B cells. If a B cell, with a related surface MHC and antigen receptor, can bind to the activated CD4+ lymphocyte it will begin to divide. B cells are further stimulated by the secreted lymphokine 'B cell differentiation factor' to undergo clonal expansion to produce genetically identical daughter cells. The daughter cells develop into either:

a. PLASMA CELLS, which actually secrete the antibody, or
b. MEMORY CELLS, which enter the circulating lymphocyte pool and persist for months/years.

Factors associated with the primary immunisation process

a. Immunoglobulin produced is predominantly IgM.
b. There is a 'lag period' of several days to several weeks, i.e. the time period between the host encountering a particular antigen and detectable antibody being found.
c. During the lag period the B cell undergoes reorganisation of genetic material, assembly of ribosomes, initiation of DNA synthesis and ultimately mitosis. If this process is disturbed, the amount of antibody produced is drastically reduced.
d. Via different signals from T cells or mutations of the B cells, the immunoglobulin produced can be either:
   • Switched from IgM to IgG, IgA, IgD or IgE
   • The same immunoglobulin type but with a higher antigen affinity
e. Some large antigenic molecules (e.g. multiple repeating polysaccharides) called 'T-cell independent antigens' can induce antibody production without the intervention of T cells (e.g. ABO, Lewis and P system glycolipids).

Secondary ('anamnestic') response
This type of response is produced by the 'primed' (memory) B lymphocytes being exposed to a second dose of the same antigen, i.e. at a time after the exposure that resulted in the primary immune response. There appears to be a need for a time delay between the two antigenic exposures for the secondary response to be produced. The secondary response is independent of T cell involvement.

In general (though not always) the secondary response results in the production of larger amounts of invariably IgG (rather than IgM) antibody, with little time delay. In addition, certain B cell clones may undergo somatic mutation and start to produce an antibody with improved affinity for the antigen, i.e. 'tailors' the antibody to produce a 'better fit' with its antigen, thereby increasing its reactivity (avidity). Generally, the decline in antibody production is slower than that seen in the primary response and may frequently continue at a high level for many years.

Regulation of the immune response
Antibody production is limited via:

a. Individual plasma cell life span (i.e. they survive for only a few days) and unless new plasma cells evolve, antibody production ceases.
b. Antibody (produced by the immune response) coats macrophage bound antigen, so that it no longer stimulates clonal expansion.
c. Suppressor T cells (CD8+) are activated, causing inhibition of further lymphocyte stimulation.
d. The antigen that initially stimulated the response may be degraded or eliminated from the body.

Antibodies to blood group antigens may be produced under the following circumstances:

1. In response to environmental antigen

Chemical structures, identical to some (especially carbohydrate) blood group antigens are very common in nature (i.e. present on the surface of bacteria and in food) and may therefore be introduced into the body independently of red cells. Antibodies are produced to these structures, which are then described as antibodies to 'red cell antigens' (i.e. because they are detectable in tests using red cells as targets).

This method accounts mainly for the production of antibodies to the A and B antigens of the ABO system, i.e. anti-A, anti-B and anti-A,B (see Section 3: The ABO blood group system), but may also result in the production of some examples of other apparent red cell antibody specificities (e.g. anti-K, anti-E, etc.). Due to the fact that these antibodies are produced in the absence of overt stimulation by foreign red cells they are often referred to by blood group serologists as either "naturally occurring" or "naturally acquired".

2. In response to a red cell antigen

The red cells from one person may be introduced into the circulation of another person by two mechanisms, transfusion or pregnancy, either of which may result in antibody formation (i.e. due to the presence of foreign red cell antigen stimulating the person's immune response). Such antibodies, if produced, are called "immune" (i.e. alloantibodies). The production of such antibodies as a result of a transfusion is however a relatively rare event, i.e. only approximately 2-9% of patients.

The basic mechanisms of immune antibody production to a red cell antigen 'X' may be demonstrated diagrammatically as follows:

a. TRANSFUSION

   X-negative recipient with an X-positive donor

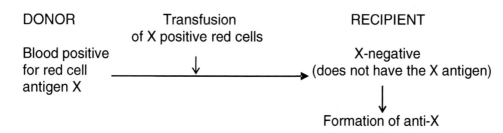

b. PREGNANCY

   X-negative woman with an X-positive partner

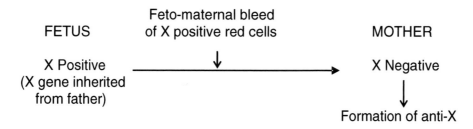

ANTIBODY STRUCTURE

An immunoglobulin molecule is composed of 'heavy' and 'light' types of protein chains, held together by non-covalent interactions and disulphide bonds. There are five possible variations of heavy chain types, i.e. gamma (G or γ), mu (M or μ), alpha (A or α), delta (D or δ) and epsilon (E or ε), which determine the five 'classes' of immunoglobulins, i.e. IgG, IgM, IgA, IgD and IgE respectively. These chain types differ in length, carbohydrate content (glycosylation), etc., resulting in each of them having different characteristics and biological activity. The gamma chain type has four variations, producing four sub-types of IgG (i.e. IgG1, IgG2, IgG3 and IgG4) that also results in variations in their biological activity. Most immune IgG blood group antibodies are of sub-types IgG1 and IgG3, and only rarely are they IgG2 or IgG4. There are two classes of IgA, i.e. IgA1 and IgA2.

There are two types of light chain, kappa (K or κ) and lambda (L or λ). The light chains of antibody molecules produced by each single clone of immunocytes will be the same types. Blood group antibodies present in serum/plasma are invariably either of the type IgG or IgM, being only rarely IgA and never IgD or IgE.

ANTIBODY CHARACTERISTICS

Basic characteristics of the immunoglobulin classes IgG and IgM

CHARACTERISTIC	IgG	IgM
Type of heavy chain	γ	μ
Type of light chain	κ or λ	κ or λ
Approximate molecular weight	160,000	900,000
Number of antigen combining sites per molecule	2	10
Normal serum concentration (mg/dl)	800 - 1,700	50 - 190
Percentage of total immunoglobulin	70 - 80%	5 - 10%

Basic properties of the immunoglobulin classes IgG and IgM

PROPERTY	IgG	IgM
Placental transfer	Yes	No
Complement activation	Yes*	Yes
Treatment with dithiothreitol (DTT)	Unaffected	Reduced
Normal reaction temperature	37°C	4°C - 20°C
Primary immune response involvement	Rare	Yes
Secondary immune response involvement	Yes	Rare

* Based on IgG binding characteristics – see Complement, Section 2

Basic properties of the IgG subclasses, related to blood group antibodies

PROPERTY	IgG1	IgG2	IgG3	IgG4
Mean percentage of total IgG	~ 70%	~ 18%	~ 8%	~ 4%
Complement activation (via the classic pathway)	++++	++	++++	+/-
Placental transfer	++++	++	++++	++
Macrophage binding	++++	++	++++	+/-

SIMPLIFIED IMMUNOGLOBULIN STRUCTURES

The two light chains and two γ heavy chains of an IgG molecule are held together by disulphide bonds between cysteine amino acids (and by non-covalent hydrophobic interactions).

Basic (simplified) structure of the IgG immunoglobulin

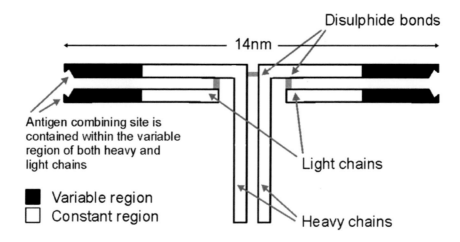

The IgM molecule is a pentameric form with the five sections, each comprising two light chains and two μ heavy chains, being held together by a J-chain.

Basic (simplified) structure of the IgM immunoglobulin

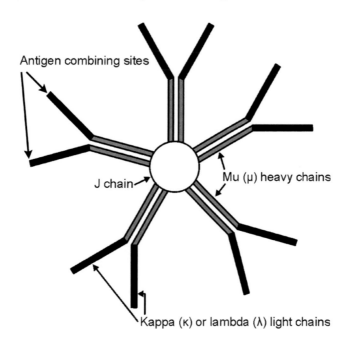

FUNCTIONAL AREAS OF IMMUNGLOBULIN MOLECULES

An IgG immunoglobulin molecule may be broken down to identify its functional areas by the use of sufficiently strong concentrations of proteolytic enzymes. At these concentrations, the action of the enzyme papain produces two Fab fragments and one Fc fragment, whereas pepsin acts to produce one F(ab')$_2$ fragment (essentially two joined Fragment Antigen Binding (Fab) fragments) and two free carboxy-terminal chains.

The Fab fragment is composed of an intact light chain and the amino-terminal end of the γ heavy chain, linked together by interchain disulphide bonding. The Fab portion has been shown to contain specific antigen binding ability, i.e. each Fab portion contains one antigen-binding site.

The Fc (Fragment Crystalline) fragment is composed of a dimer of the carboxy terminal portions of the two γ heavy chains linked by disulphide bonding and is associated with some of the IgG molecule's biological functions (e.g. complement activation and macrophage binding). The Fc fragment of the IgG molecule contains most of the carbohydrate content.

Enzyme (papain) digestion of an IgG molecule

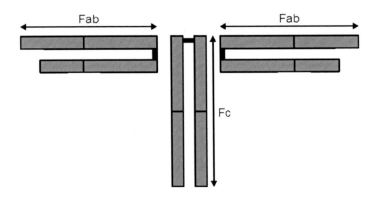

Both heavy and light chains can be divided into specific areas, which are known to have specific functions, as follows:

Variable Region
This section is at the amino-terminal end of the polypeptide chains and is approximately 110 amino acids long. It determines the specificity of the antibody and is composed of variable amino acid sequences, containing "hyper-variable" regions, which are concerned with antigen binding. This variability is generated by the immune response, which is able to generate a vast number of unique antibody specificities capable of reacting with the enormous diversity of potential antigens. For example, there are between 500-1000 heavy chain and over 200 light chain variable region genes, with the capability of producing >10 million potential specificities.

Constant Region
As the name suggests, this section of amino acids at the carboxy-terminal end of the polypeptide chain is virtually identical for a given class or sub-class of immunoglobulin. This section determines some of the biological functions of the antibody, e.g. complement activation, placental transfer and the ability to bind to effector cells (macrophages). This region also contains the immunoglobulin 'serum groups' (e.g. the Gm groups, which are genetically determined differences in the amino-acid sequence of the γ heavy chains of different IgG subtypes and between the same IgG subtype of different people).

Hinge region
This is located within the constant section of the heavy chains and centres around two closely associated triplets of proline amino acids. This region provides the heavy chain a degree of flexibility, enabling it to change its shape. An IgG molecule maintains a 'T' shape in serum/plasma enabling the antigen binding sites to be maximally distant from each other at ~14nm. The IgG immunoglobulin becomes a 'Y'

shape on binding with its antigen, which allows greater accessibility of the constant region (e.g. for complement activation).

IgG antibody structural changes related to its reaction with antigen

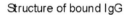

Structure of bound IgG

Structure of unbound IgG

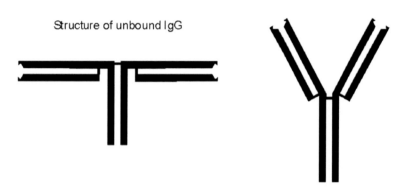

Most IgM molecules appear symmetrical, with a diameter of ~30nm. These molecules, as well as being flexible at the hinge regions of each of the individual pentameric components, change shape on binding with an antigen (like IgG molecules) and also have the capability of assuming various "crab-like" shapes due to movement at the J-chain binding sites.

Examples of possible variable structures of bound IgM molecules

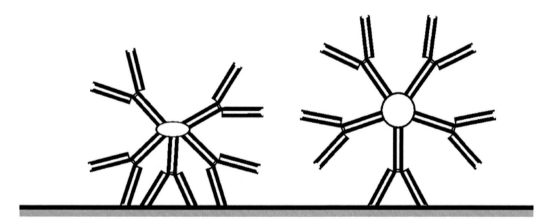

Red cell membrane - antigen structures

Domain regions
In their native states, the polypeptide chains of immunoglobulin molecules do not exist as linear sequences of amino acids but are folded, by intrachain disulphide bonds, into globular regions or domains. Extensive folding of the variable regions of both heavy and light chains brings the hyper-variable amino acid regions (which determine the antibody specificity) into close proximity to the antigen structure. This enables the immunoglobulin to form a structure to enable maximum contact with antigen.

Simplified domain structure of an IgG molecule

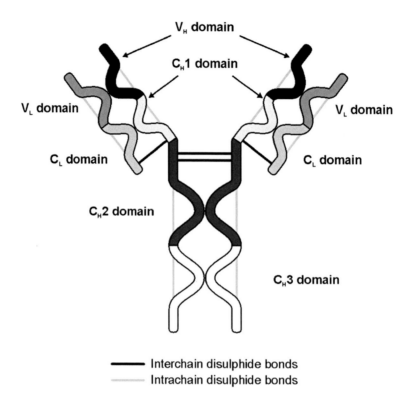

V_H domain

C_H1 domain

V_L domain

V_L domain

C_L domain

C_L domain

C_H2 domain

C_H3 domain

— Interchain disulphide bonds
— Intrachain disulphide bonds

MONOCLONAL ANTIBODIES

Many laboratory procedures now involve the use of monoclonal antibodies. These are manufactured reagents, essentially produced from (rodent or human) antibody-producing B lymphocytes that have been fused with a (myeloma) cell line or have been transformed using Epstein-Barr virus (EBV), so that the cells can be grown in culture and can therefore become 'immortal' (this is necessary since B cells die in culture). Cloning of an individual myeloma is usually done using a 'limiting dilution' technique, so that antibody production is obtained from a single cell, i.e. that secretes a single (or monoclonal) antibody specificity. Obtaining the desired antibody specificity may require numerous fusion and limiting dilution experiments and even then, this does not necessarily equate to large scale production potential.

Monoclonal antibodies are routinely used for ABO and Rh phenotyping, as well as for the grouping of a variety of other red cell antigens. Monoclonal antibodies are produced specifically to react in a 'saline room temperature' methodology, as this is easier and quicker, even though the human produced polyclonal antibody of the same specificity does not (e.g. anti-D). Monoclonal antibodies have also had a major impact on elucidating the structure of blood group antigens and the red cell membrane molecules that carry these antigens.

RED CELL AGGLUTINATION

Red cell agglutination occurs when the antigens of red cells are cross-linked by the binding of either IgG or IgM antibody molecules in a three-dimensional latticework manner, resulting in the 'clumping together' of the red cells. Red cell agglutination occurs in two distinct but inter-related stages, the antibody sensitisation (primary) stage and the agglutination (secondary) stage.

Primary stage

This 'sensitisation' stage involves the reaction of the antibody with its antigen, i.e. antibody uptake onto the red cell. Since this is a chemical reaction, it can occur very quickly and is a reversible reaction until equilibrium is reached. It is therefore governed by the Laws of Mass Action and as such is concentration dependant (i.e. increasing the concentrations of antigen and antibody produces a greater amount of antigen-antibody complex, though not as a simple linear phenomenon). The antigen and antibody are actually held together via relatively weak attracting forces, involving hydrogen, ionic and hydrophobic bonding as well as van der Waal's forces (covalent bonding is believed not to be involved in red cell antigen-antibody reactions). The major factors affecting the Primary Stage of agglutination are:

a. Red cell (antigen) to serum/plasma (antibody) ratio

The greater the amount of antibody that is present for a given amount of antigen (or conversely, the lower the red cell concentration for a given serum volume), the more antibody will become bound to its antigen. Increasing the amount of bound antibody per red cell will improve the chances of the second stage of agglutination occurring and therefore increase test sensitivity. This factor is the basis of the need to have a low concentration ('weak suspension') of red cells when performing antibody detection and/or crossmatching tests, i.e. increases the amount of antibody bound per red cell. However if the antigen concentration is very weak and the antibody concentration high (an antibody excess), few red cell aggregates are formed as most of the antigen sites are saturated with the excess of antibody as individual antibodies compete with the few antigen epitopes available. This is known as a 'prozone' effect. Conversely, an increase in the red cell concentration results in more antigen being available to react with the antibody and the amount of antibody bound per cell decreases. Although this normally results in a decrease in sensitivity (since sensitivity is dependent on the number of antibody molecules bound per red cell) this fact is utilised in the practical application of antibody adsorption techniques.

b. Ionic strength

Low Ionic Strength Saline (LISS) solution (0.03M saline with glycine added to maintain isotonicity) is designed to reduce the concentration of Na^+ and Cl^- ions per unit volume when compared with normal isotonic saline. Since the antigen and antibody molecules are themselves charged, reduction in the amount of charge in the solution between them (reducing the 'electrostatic barrier') allows the antigen-antibody reaction to occur faster. The rate of association between antigen and antibody can be speeded-up by decreasing the ionic strength of the suspending medium, since a reduction in the number of available ions in the suspending medium reduces the interfering effects of the electrostatic barrier, allowing better attraction between antigen and antibody. The use of LISS therefore frequently allows an increase in the rate of antibody uptake onto the red cell (thereby allowing a reduction of 'incubation' times).

NOTE: Although there are fewer charged ions in LISS, there is no evidence that the 'ionic cloud' surrounding a red cell in LISS is 'smaller', i.e. the red cells do not move closer together in LISS, compared with red cells in normal saline. It is the density of the ions in the 'ionic cloud' that changes. As such, LISS only affects the rate at which antibodies are able to react with red cell antigens and does not decrease the distance between individual red cells. Excessive lowering of the ionic strength of the suspending medium will result in the non-specific adherence of antibody to red cells. As such, the ionic strength of LISS and the volumes of red cells and plasma used are critical to enabling this effect to occur correctly.

c. Temperature

The nature of a particular antigen-antibody bond determines if the reaction occurs better at colder (4°C-20°C) or warmer (37°C) temperatures, i.e. exothermic antigen-antibody reactions (due to hydrogen bonds) occur better (quicker) at lower temperatures, since the heat generated during the reaction is dissipated quicker. Exothermic bonds are normally associated with carbohydrate antigens (e.g. A, B, H, Le^{a}, Le^{b}, P_{1}, I) and as a result these reactions normally proceed better at colder temperatures. Non-hydrogen bonding is normally associated with protein antigens (e.g. Rh, Kell, Duffy, etc.) and as such this type of reaction is normally optimally reactive at 37°C. From a practical viewpoint, when working with the polyclonal antibodies produced by patients, the normal reaction temperature of the different antibody specificities is governed by the nature of the antigen-antibody bond, e.g. in the laboratory ABO antibodies work best at room temperature or below, whereas Rh antibodies work best at 37°C.

Secondary stage

This involves cell to cell cross-linking by the (bivalent) antibody molecules, i.e. producing agglutination. The speed by which red cells agglutinate is determined by the frequency with which the antibody-sensitised red cells collide.

Red cells are attracted together by the action of gravity (the effects of which can be increased artificially by centrifugation) and by surface tension (i.e. interfacial energy). However, these aggregating forces are balanced by a repelling force associated with red cells having a net negative charge due to the negative charges expressed on the major membrane structure component, glycoproteins.

In suspension, the net negatively charged red cells attract a 'cloud' of (mainly) positively charged ions from the suspending saline medium. The intensity of the ionic cloud (which moves with the red cell) decreases in intensity with increasing distance from the red cell surface. This effectively produces a charged double layer. The resulting charge expressed through this cloud is known as the zeta-potential. The value of the zeta-potential dictates the minimum distance that the red cells are able to approach each other, which is therefore related to red cell surface charge density and the charged particles in the suspending medium. A number of other forces acting on the red cell membrane, including the movement of water molecules at the membrane surface are also believed to affect red cell attraction and repulsion.

The balance of the aggregating and repelling forces is such that there is a net repulsive force acting when red cells come close together, i.e. the nearest that two cells may approach is the edge of their respective ionic clouds, the so called 'slipping plane'. This repulsive force is such that the red cells cannot approach close enough to allow an IgG molecule to span the gap between them. An IgM antibody molecule is however large enough to span this gap and therefore IgM molecules are capable of causing agglutination of red cells in a saline medium. IgG antibody molecules therefore usually require an alteration to the environment of the red cells to enable them to accomplish cross-linking of red cell antigens (i.e. such as the use of enzyme treatment or the presence of anti-human globulin (AHG) reagent).

Schematic representation of factors affecting the minimum distance between red cells (not to scale)

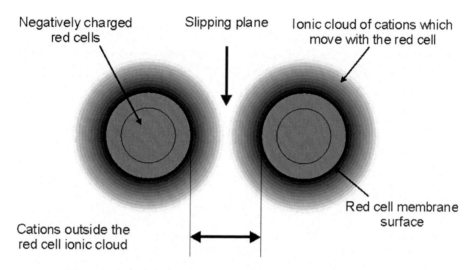

Minimum distance between red cell surfaces (>14nm)

Red cell agglutination by IgG antibodies

During the incubation phase, the red cells settle together allowing cross-linking by IgM antibody molecules. This effect can be speeded-up by the use of gentle centrifugation, which therefore enables a quicker reaction to occur. Centrifugation does not however affect agglutination by the majority of IgG antibodies as these are physically too small to span the gap between antigens on different red cells. Because of this, the second stage of agglutination of red cells by IgG antibodies requires either an alteration to the suspending environment (i.e. by the use of aggregating agents), a change to the red cell membrane charge (i.e. by the use of enzyme treatment) or the use of additional cross-linking antibodies (i.e. anti-human globulin).

a. Addition of aggregating agents

Substances such as 20% bovine albumin or polybrene (hexadimethrine bromide) effectively reduce the 'charge density' (known as the dielectric constant) of the red cell environment, thereby reducing the net repulsive force between red cells. This allows the red cells to approach closer together than is normally possible in a saline environment (causing reversible aggregation) so that some IgG antibody molecules can span the gap between red cells, producing cross-linkage and therefore agglutination. It is believed that some of these substances may also act by binding to the outer surface of the red cell membrane, affecting membrane water and therefore altering interfacial tension. This method has variable sensitivity and does not enable all IgG red antibody specificities to produce agglutination. As such is of limited practical use. Polyethylene glycol (PEG) may be employed to increase the uptake of antibody onto the red cell and is may be used in conjunction with the AHG technique.

b. Use of enzymes

Since the negative charge of a red cell is carried on the glycoprotein molecules within the red cell membrane, proteolytic enzymes (such as papain) can, when used in the correct concentration, break down and remove some of these molecules, effectively reducing the net-negative charge expressed by these red cell membrane proteins. This reduces the overall membrane charge, thereby enabling red cells to approach closer together, allowing some IgG antibody molecule specificities to produce agglutination.

Removal of some of the protein material from the red cell surface has a number of other effects, i.e. some antigenic specificities become 'more exposed' by the enzymatic removal of glycoproteins from the membrane surface and therefore generally react well with their respective antibodies by this technique (e.g. Rh). This occurs since some of the charged proteins physically close an antigen are removed (i.e. reducing what is known as 'steric hindrance'), so that the antigen becomes more accessible to an antibody. However, other antigens, which are present within glycoproteins, are destroyed by the enzyme treatment and do not therefore work by this technique (e.g. Fy^a and Fy^b antigens).

c. Anti-human globulin (AHG) technique

This technique, by the use of anti-human IgG antibody reagent, effectively cross-links IgG antibody sensitised red cells. Anti-human globulin reagent produces a 'bridging effect', where the Fab portion of the anti-human globulin antibody reacts with the Fc portion of the IgG antibody present on the (sensitised) red cells. This therefore effectively overcomes the problem of the minimum distance between red cells, which individual IgG antibodies are incapable of spanning (see Section 6: The Anti-Human Globulin Test).

Diagrammatic representation of the effect of anti-human globulin reagent (not to scale)

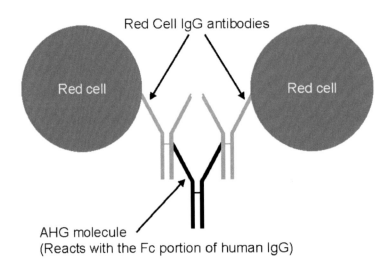

Red Cell IgG antibodies

Red cell

Red cell

AHG molecule
(Reacts with the Fc portion of human IgG)

QUESTIONS - SECTION 1

1. List the major characteristics of IgG and IgM antibodies.

2. List the main factors affecting the uptake of antibody onto red cells (i.e. sensitisation of red cells).

3. List the main factors affecting the second stage of agglutination of red cells.

4. What is an anamnestic response?

5. Why are IgG antibodies unable to agglutinate red cells in a saline medium?

6. Why should homozygous red cells be used for antibody detection?

7. Which red cell antigens are glycoprotein and which are carbohydrate?

8. How are 'naturally occurring' antibodies produced?

9. Define the terms 'antigen' and 'antibody'.

10. What is the factor that defines whether an antibody reacts best at $4^{\circ}C$-$20^{\circ}C$ or $37^{\circ}C$?

ASSIGNMENT

From your Blood Bank records, for previously untested patients, obtain the following information, which will be used in subsequent assignments:

a. Document the ABO and Rh D groups of (at least) 200 patients who have been grouped by your laboratory

b. Identify how many of these patients had a positive antibody screening test

c. Identify and document what antibody specificities were found

d. Identify the ABO and Rh D groups of the donations that were crossmatched for the patients selected.

SECTION 2

ANTIBODY MEDIATED RED CELL DESTRUCTION

Antibodies do not destroy red cells directly in the body, but initiate their destruction in two ways by:

a. The activation of complement
b. Macrophage recognition of red cell bound antibody (immune adherence)

COMPLEMENT *IN VIVO*

The 'Classical' complement pathway
The complement system is made up of nine main components (protein molecules), C1-C9. These work in a sequential manner, each one, once activated, being capable of stimulating the activation of another in a similar manner to the coagulation process. The 'classic' complement cascade is activated by the binding of one IgM molecule or two IgG molecules very close together on the red cell membrane. The order of the reaction sequence is: C1 – C4 – C2 – C3 – C5 – C6 – C7 – C8 – C9.

If the complement cascade goes to completion (C9), 'channels' are formed through the phospholipid red cell membrane at the original site of the complement activation. This allows water to move into the red cell resulting in cell lysis (haemolysis). This form of red cell destruction occurs rapidly within the circulation and is therefore termed intravascular.

The 'Classical' complement pathway can be described in three interrelated phases:

Activation phase
This involves the activation of C1 as a consequence of red cell antigen-antibody reactions, together with the subsequent activation of C4 and C2 molecules.

The C1 molecule is composed of three sub-units, C1q, C1r and C1s and is activated by an antigen-antibody reaction. Calcium ions are essential for the integrity of the C1 molecule and strong calcium chelating agents, such as ethylene-diamine-tetra-acetic acid (EDTA) and citrate anticoagulants will disrupt the C1 molecule and inhibit complement activation. Therefore if plasma is used instead of serum in serological reactions the C1 molecule will be disrupted. As a result complement will not be activated and cannot therefore be detected by the anti-human globulin (AHG) technique.

The C1q portion of the C1 molecule contains six immunoglobulin-binding sites, which enables the intact C1 molecule to bind to the C_H2 domain of the Fc portion of principally IgG1, IgG3 or IgM antigen-bound immunoglobulins.

Binding to two Fc portions of IgG activates C1q. This does not occur unless two IgG antibody molecules are bound to the red cell membrane in close proximity, within <40nm of each other, or by a single IgM immunoglobulin molecule, as each molecule has five available Fc binding sites. To enable this binding to occur, it has been calculated that approximately 800 antibody molecules would have to bind to a single red cell expressing 600,000 evenly spaced antigen sites of a particular specificity, so as to provide a single potential C1q activation site. This requirement acts as a restriction to complement activation and may be further affected by the low numbers or non-random distribution of some antigen sites on the red cell membrane surface. This factor alone probably explains why some blood group antibodies (e.g. Rh antibodies), which although

IgG1 and/or IgG3, and therefore theoretically capable of doing so, do not activate complement.

The binding of C1q with the Fc portions of two IgG or one IgM red cell membrane bound immunoglobulin antibody molecules activates the C1 molecule. Activated C1 then acts simultaneously on C4 and C2 molecules. The C4 molecule is cleaved into two components C4a, which is released into the fluid phase, and C4b which binds covalently with the Fc region of the red cell bound immunoglobulin or to the cell membrane itself, around the C1 site.

The C2 molecule is also cleaved by activated C1 into two components, C2a, which is released into the fluid phase and C2b which, in the presence of Ca^{++}, binds onto C4b forming C4b2b complexes (known as 'C3 convertase'). Numerous C4b and C2b complexes are produced by the action of a single activated C1 molecule, and these are bound around a single C1 activation site, therefore acting to amplify the effect.

The activation of C4 and C2 may however be inhibited by either a C1 inhibitor protein (C1 INH) or by the short half-life of the active C2b molecule (i.e. this molecule quickly inactivates and the C4b2b complex rapidly dissociates).

Schematic diagram of the activation of C4 and C2 by activated C1

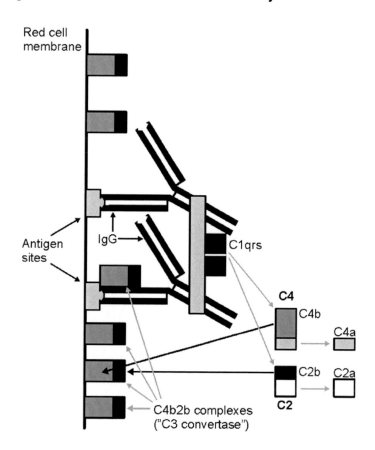

Amplification phase

This involves the activation of C3 by the activated C4b2b complex ('C3 convertase'), resulting in the binding of C3b onto this complex, as well as to numerous other sites on the red cell membrane.

Once formed, the C4b2b complex activates the C3 molecule, breaking it into two components. The smaller fragment (C3a) is released into the fluid phase and acts as an anaphylatoxin (see below) causing increased vascular permeability. The larger fragment (C3b) is bound to the C4b2b complex, producing a single C4b2b3b complex. This in turn is capable of activating numerous other C3 molecules, which become bound to the red cell membrane (approximately 100 C3b molecules are bound for each C4b2b complex produced). This is a major amplification stage of the classic complement activation sequence.

This stage can also however be inactivated by either the short half life of the C3b molecule which rapidly inactivates if it is not bound immediately to the cell membrane, or by the action of C3b and/or C4b inactivator proteins (C3bINA and C4bINA respectively). Because of the action of these control molecules and/or regulatory mechanisms, the complement cascade frequently stops at the C3b stage.

The binding of C3b onto the membrane surface confers the red cell with immune adherence properties, in that the red cell becomes capable of being bound by specific C3b receptor sites on macrophages. As a result, these C3b coated red cells are removed from the circulation and since the macrophages are tissue bound, mainly within the liver, this type of red cell destruction is termed extravascular (see below). However, the red cell bound C3b may be inactivated by a C3bINA protein and as macrophages have no receptor for this inactive form of C3 (C3d), these complement coated red cells have a near normal life span. A positive reaction using an anti-C3d AHG reagent with DAT positive red cells therefore provides evidence that complement activation has taken place in the patient's circulation.

Schematic diagram of the activation of C3 by activated C4b2b

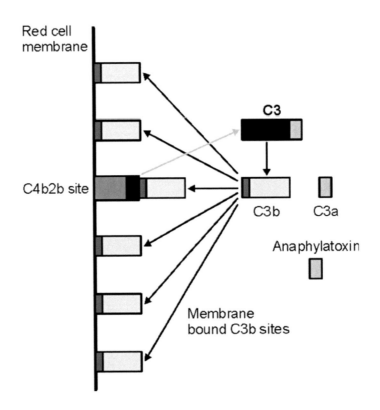

Membrane attack phase
This involves the activation of C5 by the C4b2b3b complex and the subsequent activation of C6, C7, C8 and C9.

Each C4b2b3b complex is capable of activating a C5 molecule, which is cleaved into two components. The smaller C5a fragment, which is released into the fluid phase, acts as an anaphylatoxin (causes increased vascular permeability – see below) and also as a chemotactic factor (causes the directed migration of polymorphonuclear leucocytes). The C5b molecule is bound to the red cell membrane and is then capable of activating a C6 as well as a C7 molecule, which are both bound to the C5b molecule, forming a stable tri-molecular complex that becomes firmly inserted into the phospholipid bi-layer of the membrane. One C8 and between 10-16 C9 molecules are then bound to each activated C5b67 site in a circular manner to form a tubular structure. When activated and bound in this way, these terminal components produce a membrane lesion or hole, which is approximately 10nm in diameter. This allows the free movement of ions and water across the membrane, rapidly resulting in the loss of osmotic gradient and red cell lysis.

The 'Classical' complement pathway

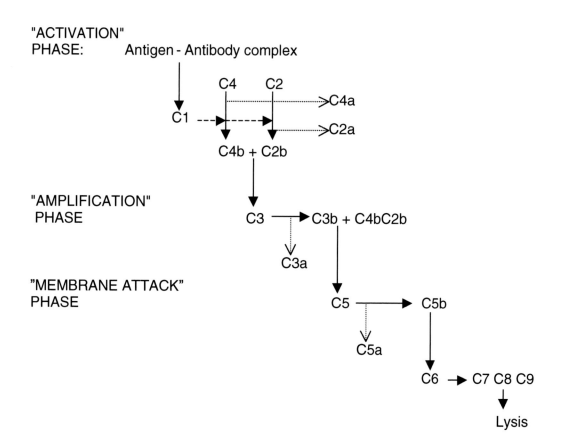

COMPLEMENT *IN VITRO*

If a serum sample is used in the laboratory, antigen-antibody reactions may activate complement causing the binding of C3 onto the red cell membrane, which may subsequently be detected in the anti-human globulin (AHG) test, or the red cells may be lysed if the complement pathway goes to completion. Therefore, lysis should be noted as a positive reaction when reading tests.

Complement can be inactivated by either heat (e.g. $56^{\circ}C$ for 30 minutes) since C1 and C2 are heat labile, or by the presence of calcium binding anticoagulants (e.g. EDTA and citrate), due to the fact that the C1 molecule structure is dependant upon the presence of free calcium ions. As a result, antibodies present in plasma, as opposed to serum, will not produce either lysis or the binding of C3 to red cells, which therefore cannot be detected in laboratory AHG tests.

'Broad spectrum' AHG reagents (which contain both anti-C3 and anti-IgG) were developed to detect both IgG and C3 bound to the red cell. This was believed to improve the sensitivity of the AHG test. The use of a 'broad spectrum' AHG reagent is therefore of limited use when used with the anticoagulated (plasma) samples, required by the automated equipment used in transfusion laboratories. However, it is also debatable how useful the detection of both C3 and IgG is, since weak alloantibodies are frequently incapable of activating complement (see Section 7: Antibody Detection and Identification).

RED CELL DESTRUCTION *IN VIVO*

Intravascular Lysis
When an antigen-antibody reaction results in complement activation with the sequence going to completion, the red cell membranes are damaged and lyse within the circulation. This releases haemoglobin into the blood stream leading to haemoglobinaemia and haemoglobinuria. Examples of antibodies, which are haemolytic *in vivo*, are mainly anti-A, anti-B and particularly anti-A,B. Since most deaths resulting from the transfusion of incompatible blood are associated with strongly lytic antibodies, ABO incompatibility is of prime importance.

Extravascular Lysis
Apart from anti-A, anti-B and anti-A,B most other antibody specificities bring about red cell destruction by macrophages outside the circulation, i.e. extravascular. Not all IgG and IgM antibodies activate complement; Rh antibodies for instance do not. When such IgG antibody molecules bind to red cells *in vivo* in the absence of complement activation the bound IgG is recognised by macrophage IgG receptors (FcγR). However, macrophage IgG receptors also react with free, unbound, IgG and therefore, the binding of IgG coated red cells to macrophages only occurs in areas of the body where the amount of free plasma and therefore IgG is low, principally in the spleen. The red cells are then either engulfed by the macrophage or a part of the membrane is removed allowing the rest of the red cell to break away as a spherocyte, which are subsequently trapped in the microcirculation of the spleen. Macrophage C3b receptors are not inhibited by free C3 and therefore red cells coated with C3b (see above) are recognised and removed principally by macrophages in the liver. Red cells coated with both IgG and C3b can be removed in either the spleen and/or the liver. The rate of destruction depends on a number of factors such as the amount of antibody bound per red cell and the number of (incompatible) antibody coated red cells present, but this destruction can be rapid enough to produce some haemoglobinuria.

CLINICAL EFFECTS OF *IN VIVO* RED CELL DESTRUCTION

The clinical signs and symptoms of *in vivo* red cell destruction such as those seen in a haemolytic transfusion reaction might include some (or all) of the following:

- Fever (>1°C rise in temp)
- Flushing of the face
- Chest pain
- Lumbar pain
- Hypotension
- Nausea

In extreme cases:

- Haemoglobinuria
- Anuria – renal damage
- Unexplained bleeding – Disseminated Intravascular Coagulation (DIC)

Anaphylatoxins

These symptoms can be largely explained by the anaphylactic and chemotactic action of C5a and C3a molecules, which are released into the plasma during complement activation. In addition, pro-inflammatory cytokines such as tumour necrosis factor (TNF) and interleukin-1 (IL-1) are also activated. These cytokines can cause hypotension, may activate the fibrinolytic pathway leading to DIC or cause the renal circulation to be reduced, hence renal failure (see Section 9: Transfusion Reactions).

Management of an acute haemolytic transfusion reaction includes maintaining a good fluid balance by infusing saline to support kidney function, and replacing coagulation factors or platelets in cases of DIC by transfusing platelet concentrates and fresh frozen plasma (FFP).

CLINICAL SIGNIFICANCE OF ANTIBODIES

Not all red cell alloantibodies are capable of causing red cell destruction *in vivo*. There are a number of factors which contribute to the destructive potential of an antibody, including:

- Immunoglobulin class
- IgG sub-class
- Blood group antigen specificity
- Complement activation
- Activity at 37°C

However, those antibodies that are reactive at 37°C by an antiglobulin test are generally considered to be 'clinically significant' (see Section 7: Antibody Detection and Identification). Clinically significant antibodies are capable of causing a transfusion reaction (incompatible red cell destruction) and/or Haemolytic Disease of the Fetus/ Newborn (HDFN) (see Section 8: Pre-Transfusion Testing, Section 11: Haemolytic Disease of the Fetus/Newborn, and Section 12: Immune Haemolytic Anaemias).

QUESTIONS - SECTION 2

1. Explain intravascular red cell removal.

2. Explain extravascular red cell removal.

3. How are red cells removed by macrophages in the liver and spleen?

4. What activates the classic complement pathway?

5. Why is complement not able to be activated *in vitro* using anticoagulated (plasma) samples?

6. Identify the three phases of the classic complement pathway

7. How many IgG or IgM antibody molecules are required to activate C1?

8. What clinical effects define an antibody as 'clinically significant'?

9. How do 'clinically significant' antibodies react *in vitro*?

10. How is complement inactivated?

SECTION 3

THE ABO BLOOD GROUP SYSTEM

The ABO system was described in 1901 by Karl Landsteiner and was the first blood group system to be discovered. It is by far the most important blood group system in transfusion due to the fact that antibodies are always present in a person's serum/plasma against antigens not present on their red cells. This is the basis of Landsteiner's Law, which states:

'Whenever an (A and/or B) antigen is not present on the red cells, the corresponding antibody is found in the serum'.

These antibodies are produced as a result of environmental stimulation and are capable of producing intravascular haemolysis, i.e. the destruction of incompatible red cells in the person's circulation, via complement activation (see Section 2: Antibody Mediated Red Cell Destruction).

ABO is by far the most clinically important blood group system in transfusion. This is due to the following combination of factors:

- The (environmentally stimulated) antibodies are always present in a healthy person's plasma when the person lacks the corresponding antigen. Therefore the vast majority of the general population (i.e. everyone but group AB and therefore approximately 97% of people in the UK) have either anti-A, anti-B or anti-A,B present in their serum/plasma.
- The nature of ABO antibodies, in that they are capable of producing intravascular haemolysis of incompatible red cells via complement activation.
- The very high frequency of A and/or B antigens in the general population (i.e. approximately 55% in the UK), together with the high density of antigens per red cell when present.

Almost all reported serious / fatal transfusion reactions, caused by either clerical or technical error, are the result of ABO blood group incompatibility. This illustrates the enormous clinical importance of the ABO blood group system.

ABO GROUPS AND THEIR FREQUENCIES

GROUP	UK FREQUENCY (approximate)	ANTIGENS PRESENT ON THE RED CELLS	ANTIBODIES PRESENT IN THE PLASMA
A	43%	A	Anti-B
B	9%	B	Anti-A
O	45%	None (H)	Anti-A,B
AB	3%	A and B	None

The ABO blood group genes exhibit various racial and population variations. Numerous races and peoples have been studied for their ABO gene frequencies. Black populations generally have a high incidence of group B whilst Arabs have a high incidence of group O. The ABO blood group frequencies vary slightly within the UK, i.e. group O frequency increases to the North, whereas the group A frequency increases towards the South.

MANUAL ABO GROUPING

The pre-transfusion testing guidelines identify that ABO grouping is performed:

1. Using a sample of the patient's red cells reacted against known monoclonal anti-A and anti-B grouping antisera. This is known as the "cell" group. This test is used to identify the antigens present on the patient's red cells.

2. Using the patient's serum/plasma reacted against group A and B red cells (as well as frequently group O). This is known as either the "serum" or "reverse" group. This test is used to identify the ABO antibody specificities present in the patient's serum/plasma.

Red cell reactions with		Plasma reactions with group		Red cell phenotype	Antibody present in the plasma
Anti-A	**Anti-B**	**A RBCs**	**B RBCs**		
-	-	+	+	O	Anti-A,B
+	-	-	+	A	Anti-B
-	+	+	-	B	Anti-A
+	+	-	-	AB	None

The presence of ABO antibodies in the serum/plasma of adults, which does not occur in any other blood group system, allows these two methods to be routinely used together for ABO grouping. This 'complementary testing' regime is performed to reduce the possibility of error and reflects the importance of ensuring that the ABO group is correctly ascertained, as well as enabling rarer / unusual ABO groups to be identified.

The results obtained for an ABO test should reflect the 'complementary' results identified in the above table. If anything other than the expected results are obtained, the problem should be resolved, initially by repeat grouping and if necessary by the testing of a further blood sample. The cell group result should not be taken on its own to represent the group of the patient if the serum/plasma group result obtained differs from that expected. Abnormal grouping results must be recorded and the reason why they have occurred should be investigated. A number of circumstances may give rise to anomalous ABO grouping results (see below).

THE CONCEPT OF "UNIVERSAL DONOR - UNIVERSAL RECIPIENT"

Due to the absence of antigens on the red cells of a group O and the absence of antibodies in the serum/plasma of a group AB, these groups were termed "universal donor" and "universal recipient" respectively. This practice is no longer followed, the current practice being to transfuse blood only of the same ABO group as the recipient whenever possible.

RECIPIENT	DONOR
A	A (O)
B	B (O)
O	O
AB	AB (A, B or O)

Only in exceptional circumstances should group AB recipients be transfused with the red cells of either group A, B or O; or group O red cells be given to any non-group O recipient (see also ABO antibodies - below).

ABO ANTIBODIES

ABO antibodies are described as being "naturally acquired" because they are present in the serum of all healthy adults. In reality, these antibodies are produced in response to stimulation from environmental (e.g. bacterial and viral) material (see Section 1: Antigen-antibody reactions). Children under 3 months usually have little or no antibody present in their serum/plasma due to their underdeveloped immune system and lack of antigenic exposure. Any antibody present in a baby's serum/plasma at birth is likely to be of maternal origin, resulting from placental transfer of IgG antibody. In addition, ABO antigens may be only weakly expressed at birth. Antibody strength reaches normal adult levels at approximately 5 years of age, remains relatively stable during adult life and then usually declines in old age. The routine presence of antibodies in the serum/plasma is unique to the ABO system.

Anti-A,B produced by group O people is a single antibody capable of reacting with either the A or B antigen and is not the same as anti-A+anti-B (written as anti-A+B), which is a mixture of two separate antibody specificities (i.e. produced by mixing the anti-A from a group B and the anti-B from a group A). Some group O individuals have extremely strong ('high titre') anti-A,B that is capable, via complement activation, of lysing red cells *in vitro* (in the laboratory) as well as *in vivo* (in the body). These haemolytic antibodies could cause problems in people of other ABO groups if transfused in a large enough volume, especially if transfused to babies or children who have a small blood volume.

ABO GENETICS

The ABO genetic locus is situated on chromosome number 9. Basically, one of three allelic gene options may be present at this genetic locus, the *A* gene, *B* gene or *O* gene (Note: italics are used in text to identify a gene). The *O* gene produces no antigenic product (is therefore said to be amorphic) and is recessive to both *A* and *B* genes (which are co-dominant). Since each individual has a pair of number 9 chromosomes (i.e. inherits two ABO genes, one paternal and one maternal in origin), they together produce the person's ABO genotype, which determines their ABO group. Therefore the possible gene combinations are:

BLOOD GROUP	RED CELL ANTIGENS (PHENOTYPE)	GENES PRESENT (POSSIBLE GENOTYPES)
A	A	*AA* or *AO*
B	B	*BB* or *BO*
O	None	*OO*
AB	A and B	*AB*

Therefore, although there are 6 possible genotype combinations, because the *O* gene is recessive (or amorphic) there are only 4 phenotypes. The phenotype therefore represents the antigens expressed on the red cells and the genotype is the genes that produce them. The group O phenotype can therefore only be produced by an *OO* genotype and similarly the AB phenotype by an *AB* genotype. The group A phenotype can be produced by either of the genotypes *AA* or *AO* and likewise the B phenotype by the genotypes *BB* or *BO*.

The ABO antigens do not show 'dosage effects', i.e. although the presence of two identical genes results in the production of more antigens per red cell, a group A person's red cells produced by the (homozygote) *AA* genotype do not react more strongly with anti-A than the group A red cells of the (heterozygote) *AO* genotype. The only way therefore to distinguish the difference between the genotypes *AA/AO* and *BB/BO* is by informative family studies or by the use of molecular genetic (DNA analysis) techniques to detect the relevant genes.

ABO INHERITANCE - EXAMPLES

PARENTS
     Phenotype   :   O   x   AB
     Genotype   :   *OO*   *AB*

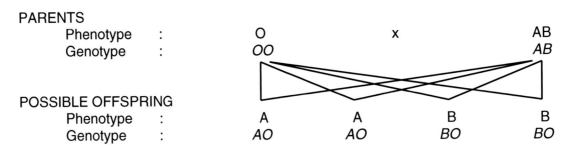

POSSIBLE OFFSPRING
     Phenotype   :   A   A   B   B
     Genotype   :   *AO*   *AO*   *BO*   *BO*

i.e. each group A or B offspring has a 50% chance of being produced.

PARENTS
     Phenotype   :   A   x   B
     Genotype   :   *AO*   *BO*

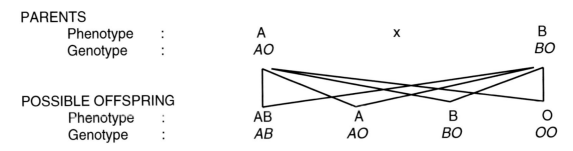

POSSIBLE OFFSPRING
     Phenotype   :   AB   A   B   O
     Genotype   :   *AB*   *AO*   *BO*   *OO*

i.e. all 4 phenotypes are possible, each with a 25% chance of being produced.

SUB-GROUPS OF GROUP A

Group A can be further divided into two main sub-groups called A_1 and A_2. Individuals of group A_2 have less A antigen sites on each of their red cells (~250,000 per cell) compared with group A_1 individuals (~1,000,000 per cell). Results of work performed on the transferase enzymes produced the A^1 and A^2 genes have shown that the enzyme produced by group A_2 people is less effective than the enzyme produced by the A^1 gene in converting H substance into A antigen, and hence fewer antigen sites are produced (see ABO genetic pathway - below). This work has been verified by DNA studies of the genes from A^1 and A^2 individuals.

Some A_2 individuals (~2%) and more frequently A_2B people (~25%), produce a 'naturally occurring' anti-A_1 antibody, which reacts with group A_1 red cells but not group A_2 red cells. This defies Landsteiner's Law, since the antibody is effectively directed against an antigen which the person has, albeit in smaller number. Anti-A_1 is however only reactive at low temperatures and is not normally reactive at $37^{\circ}C$, and as such is therefore not clinically significant. This situation is reflected in some other blood group systems, for example, many people have anti-I in their serum/plasma but all people, except very rare individuals, have the I antigen on their red cells. Anti-I is also a cold reacting antibody of no clinical significance, except in some pathological conditions. As such, this antibody may be detected when ABO grouping, in which case it is capable of reacting with all red cells used in the 'reverse group'.

The A^1 gene is dominant to the A^2 gene. Both A^1 and A^2 genes are co-dominant when present with a B gene and both are dominant when present with an O gene. Therefore, the phenotype A₁ may be produced by the A^1A^1, A^1A^2 or A^1O genotypes, whereas the phenotype A₂ results from the presence of either the A^2A^2 or A^2O genotypes. Group AB people may also be sub-divided into group A₁B and A₂B. This extends the phenotype possibilities from four to six and the possible genotypes from six to ten.

Summary of the possible genotypes producing the different ABO phenotypes

GROUP	PHENOTYPE	POSSIBLE GENOTYPE
O	O	OO
A	A₁	A^1A^1 A^1A^2 A^1O
	A₂	A^2A^2 A^2O
B	B	BB BO
AB	A₁B	A^1B
	A₂B	A^2B

ABO ANTIGEN PRODUCTION

A and B antigens are carbohydrate structures, The A and B genes determine the production of specific transferase enzymes, which act on a particular substrate (precursor substance) converting it into a specific product (antigen), i.e.

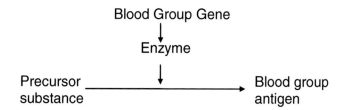

In the case of ABO, the production of the precursor substance is itself determined by the presence of another blood group gene (i.e. H). The production of the red cell A and/or B antigens is therefore dependant upon the presence of an H gene, as well as the A and/or B genes. The H and ABO genetic loci are not linked and H and ABO represent separate, though related, blood groups. It is therefore incorrect to refer to the "ABH blood group system".

The 'precursor substance' is a carbohydrate chain, present on all red cells. The presence of an H gene (either expressed as the homozygote HH or heterozygote Hh) produces the H enzyme, which causes a precursor substance to be converted into H substance, by the addition of a single terminal carbohydrate (sugar) molecule (L-fucose). The A and/or B genes, via their enzyme products, each add a further different terminal carbohydrate molecule to H substance, converting H into either A and/or B antigens. The presence of the *OO* genotype therefore means that the H substance is left unchanged.

In the absence of an *H* gene (genotype *hh*) the precursor substance remains unchanged and no H substance is produced. Since H substance is the substrate for the A and/or B enzymes, no A and/or B antigens can therefore be produced (even though the *A* and/or *B* genes are present). This rare condition, i.e. the total absence of A, B and H antigens, is known as the O_h or "Bombay" phenotype. Group O_h people routinely produce 'naturally occurring' anti-H, as well as anti-A,B, both of which are clinically significant. Indeed, it is the presence of unexpected reactions in the reverse group due to the anti-H that is usually the first indication of this rare blood group. Although the phenotype is more frequently encountered in people of the Indian sub-continent, the Bombay phenotype has been identified in many other populations.

The *A* and/or *B* genes inherited by a group O_h person, though not expressed, are capable of being transmitted normally to offspring. If, via family studies or enzyme analysis, the ABO genes present in a Bombay person is known, their phenotype may be written so as to identify this, e.g. as O_h^O, O_h^B, O_h^A, O_h^{AB}.

Bombay inheritance (example)

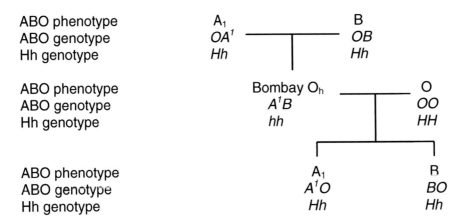

ABO phenotype	A_1	B
ABO genotype	OA^1	OB
Hh genotype	Hh	Hh

ABO phenotype	Bombay O_h	O
ABO genotype	A^1B	OO
Hh genotype	hh	HH

ABO phenotype	A_1	B
ABO genotype	A^1O	BO
Hh genotype	Hh	Hh

THE ABO GENETIC PATHWAY

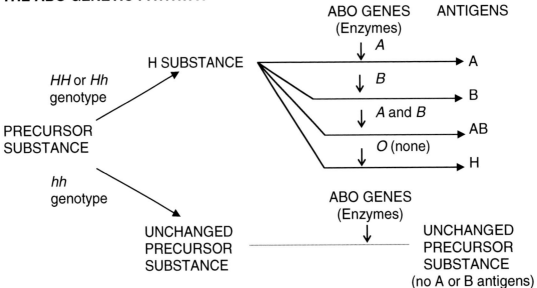

Since group O represents an amorphic gene expression, the H antigen remains 'unchanged', and is therefore present in maximal amounts on group O red cells. Groups A, B and AB have little H antigen presence, having converted most of it to either A and/or B antigen. When both *A* and *B* genes are present (group AB), almost all of the H substance is converted. The H genetic locus (chromosome 19) is independent of the ABO genetic locus (chromosome 9); therefore H and ABO represent separate, though associated, blood groups. The enzyme produced by the A^1 gene is more effective at converting H substance than is the enzyme produced by the A^2 gene. Therefore, A_2 individuals have less A antigen but more H on their red cells than A_1 people.

The H, A and B antigens are produced from a 'precursor substance' carbohydrate chain, which is itself attached to a lipid (as glycolipid) cell membrane structure. The ABH antigens are present on almost all cells of the body. The antigens are also present (as glycoprotein) in the serum/plasma. Because of this, red cells should be washed, or at least suspended, in saline before blood grouping is attempted, to avoid these soluble serum/plasma antigens from possibly inhibiting the test (grouping) antisera.

Some group A_1 and A_1B people produce anti-H which, unlike the antibody produced by O_h people, is a cold reacting clinically insignificant antibody, possibly detected during ABO grouping (i.e. in the 'reverse' or 'serum' group). Anti-H reacts most strongly with the group O red cell sample (i.e. since these express the maximal amount of H substance) and weaker with A_2, B and A_1 cells as shown below:

$\Rightarrow$ Decreasing quantities of H antigen on the red cell

GROUP: O $\Rightarrow$ A_2 $\Rightarrow$ B $\Rightarrow$ A_1 $\Rightarrow$ A_1B

The chemical structure of the H, A and B antigens was first described in 1960. The different ABH specificities are dependent upon the inheritance of the individual genes that code for specific transferase enzymes, which add specific carbohydrates to the terminal D-galactose sugar of a carbohydrate chain.

GENE	GENE PRODUCT	CARBOHYDRATE
H	α-2-L-fucosyltransferase	L-fucose
A	α-3-N-acetyl-D-galactosaminyltransferase	N-acetyl-D-galactosamine
B	α-3-D-galactosaminyltransferase	D-galactose

The ABO blood group antigenic specificities reside in the terminal carbohydrate of red cell glycolipid molecules and can be illustrated, at a basic level, as follows:

PRECURSOR SUBSTANCE :   X -- Gal -- GlcNAc -- Gal

H SUBSTANCE: X -- Gal -- GlcNAc -- Gal
                                                 |
                                               Fuc

A SUBSTANCE: X -- Gal -- GlcNAc -- Gal **-- GalNAc**
                                                 |
                                               Fuc

B SUBSTANCE: X -- Gal -- GlcNAc -- Gal **-- Gal**
                                                 |
                                               Fuc

Abbreviations used for structures in the above diagrams:

X : represents a long (branched) carbohydrate chain either attached to lipid (red cell glycolipid) or protein (secreted glycoprotein).
GalNAc : N-acetyl-D-galactosamine
GlcNAc : N-acetyl-D-glucosamine
Fuc : L-fucose
Gal : D-galactose

OTHER SUB-GROUPS OF GROUP A AND GROUP B

Various other sub-groups of group A and B exist, caused by genetic variations that result in weaker and variable reacting antigenic types, but these are rare in the UK.

Group A_3
Has a frequency of approximately 1 in 1,000 of group A people. Classically, group A_3 is identified as giving a 'mixed-field' reaction (small agglutinates in a field of un-agglutinated cells) with polyclonal anti-A and anti-A,B antisera. Monoclonal anti-A may give a weaker non mixed-field reaction with A_3 red cells. This effect is due to the low number of A antigen sites per red cell of a group A_3. Potent monoclonal antisera usually give strong (complete) agglutination with group A_3 red cells. Group A_3 people produce normal anti-B and occasionally produce anti-A_1.

Group A_x (or A_4)
Blood group A_x individuals are very rare, having a frequency of from 1 in 40,000 to 1 in 77,000 of group A people. Group A_x individuals have very few A antigen sites on their red cells, which as a result, are only agglutinated by some potent monoclonal anti-A sera and/or selected anti-A,B sera. Classically A_x red cells are not agglutinated by polyclonal anti-A but react with polyclonal anti-A,B sera but some monoclonal anti-A reagents may give a very weak reaction with A_x red cells. Group A_x people produce normal anti-B and also frequently anti-A_1 but not anti-A.

Reaction summary of group A sub-types

RED CELL PHENOTYPE	RED CELL REACTION WITH POLYCLONAL ANTISERA				PLASMA REACTION WITH RED CELLS			
	Anti-A	Anti-B	Anti-A,B	Anti-A_1	A_1	A_2	B	O
A_1	4	0	4	3	0	0	3	0
A_2	4	0	4	0	+/-	0	3	0
A_3	2mf	0	2mf	0	+/-	0	3	0
A_x (or A_4)	1*	0	2	0	1*	0	3	0

Notes:
0 = negative; 1 to 4 = increasing strengths of agglutination (positive reactions)
mf : Mixed field agglutination
+/- : Positive or negative result possible; i.e. groups A_2 and A_3 may or may not produce anti-A_1
1* : For explanation see text above

As with the A_2 phenotype, the groups A_3 and A_x are not expressed when in combination with an A^1 (or A^2) gene.

Rare sub-groups of group B also occur, but these are usually found only in Chinese and African populations, where the group B frequency is higher. In the presence of normal A (or B) genes, the genes producing these rare A (or B) phenotypes are not expressed / identified.

Acquired B

As its name suggests, this condition essentially means that a group A person appears to 'change their blood group' and become a group AB. This effect is caused by the enzymic breakdown of the group A antigen (N-acetyl-D-galactosamine) to galactosamine, which is similar enough in structure to the B antigen immunodominant sugar (D-galactose) to react with some anti-B (polyclonal and monoclonal) antisera. This antigenic change is brought about by the action of deactylase enzymes produced by some bacteria on the group A antigen (usually group A_1). The condition can occur either *in vivo* (usually associated with gastrointestinal bacterial diseases) or *in vitro* (due to blood sample bacterial infection). Monoclonal anti-B reagents used for blood grouping in the UK should not react with the acquired B antigen.

ANOMALOUS ABO GROUPING RESULTS

Occasionally when ABO typing, odd reactions that do not fit into the expected pattern are found; these should be recorded and the reason why they have occurred should be investigated. They may be due to a technical error but there are other reasons to explain most unexpected reactions. The first thing to do in such cases is to repeat the tests to ensure the reactions are genuine. If possible additional reagents, such as anti-A,B and A_2 cells, should be used, as well as the patient's own cells together with their own serum/plasma (auto control), if these are not part of the routine testing procedure. ABO anomalies fall into four broad categories:

'Additional antigens'
Additional unexpected positive reactions with anti-A or anti-B are very rare when using monoclonal grouping reagents but include:
- Acquired B (see above)
- Cells sensitised with another antibody

'Missing antigens'
Unexpected negative reactions with anti-A or anti-B or very weak expression of antigens is sometimes found in:
- Some malignant diseases such as leukaemia, where ABO antigens may become very weak or even disappear, only to return to normal during disease remission
- Red cells from a fetus or newborn infant who has poorly developed ABO antigens (these are usually detectable with most monoclonal reagents)
- An infant who has received intrauterine transfusions (IUT). As group O blood is usually used for IUT, they may appear to be group O and not their expected group

'Additional antibodies'
Unexpected positive reactions with A and/or B cells are the most common cause of anomalous reactions. These are normally due to the presence of cold reacting antibodies such as anti-P_1 or anti-I in the patient's serum/plasma. Anti-P_1 will agglutinate the A and/or B cells if they happen to carry the P_1 antigen. As all adult cells carry the I antigen, the presence of anti-I, a cold reacting autoantibody, will result in the patient's serum/plasma reacting with their own cells as well as the reagent A and B cells, but should not react at 37°C. Group A_1 or AB people can have anti-H/HI present that reacts strongly with group O cells and slightly weaker with A_2 cells, but not with A_1 cells (due to the decreasing amount of H antigen on these red cells (see above section on ABO antigen production). Repeating the test at 37°C will usually resolve the problem as the cold reactive antibodies will not react at 37°C but the anti-A/B in the patient's serum/plasma will (though a longer incubation time may be

required). Anti-A$_1$ is sometimes found in A$_2$ or more likely in A$_2$B or A$_x$ individuals; testing the serum/plasma with A$_2$ cells will confirm its specificity.

'Missing antibodies'
Unexpected negative reactions with A and/or B cells can, as with missing antigens, also occur in some disease states, but may also result from the patient's age (i.e. either very young or old – see 'ABO antibodies' earlier in this section). It can also be seen in patients who have low levels of IgM immunoglobulins or in post-bone marrow transplant (BMT) patients.

Mixed Field Reactions
Mixed field reactions, i.e. the presence of a mixture of agglutinated and unagglutinated cells, can be found in a number of situations such as:

- Post transfusion (e.g. of group O blood into a group A patient)
- Post-bone marrow transplant (e.g. group O donor BMT to a group A recipient)
- Weak expression of A or B antigen
- Rare individuals with a genetic abnormality (e.g. chimerism)
- In some diseases (e.g. leukaemia)

The mixed field reactions should be noted (i.e. by the letters mf) and when interpreting the results the patient's clinical condition and transfusion history should be taken into account.

In cases where the ABO group cannot be determined, or an unexplained mixed-field reaction found, a sample should be sent to a reference laboratory for further testing. If blood is urgently needed then group O blood, that is compatible when crossmatched by an antiglobulin technique at 37°C, can be used.

QUESTIONS - SECTION 3

1. Tabulate the expected reactions of the four ABO blood groups with anti-A, anti-B, anti-A,B together with A_1, A_2, B and O red cells.

2. Tabulate the controls you would use for routine manual ABO grouping and their expected reactions.

3. What are the possible ABO genotypes of the offspring from the following matings?

   a. Group B x Group AB
   b. Group B x Group A_2
   c. Group B x Group A_1

4. What possible genotypes produce the A_1; A_2; A_3 and A_x phenotypes?

5. Which ABO blood group has the most H substance and which has the least?

6. Anti-A_1 can be produced by which of the A subgroups?

7. Why is the ABO blood group system the most clinically important?

8. Tabulate the expected reactions of a group O and a group O_h person.

9. What are the approximate frequencies of each of the ABO blood groups in the UK?

10. What chemical structures comprise the ABO antigens?

ASSIGNMENT

Using the data collected from your Blood Bank records, calculate the frequencies of the ABO blood groups of the patients tested and donations cross-matched.

Is there a significant difference between them, and if so, can you suggest why?

ABO DATA INTERPRETATION - SECTION 3

The following table represents the ABO blood grouping results from testing 10 different patient's blood samples. All reagents and techniques have been checked and are working correctly (i.e. the results depicted are not the result of clerical or technical error). All control results are as expected.

1. Provide an ABO blood group (phenotype) interpretation of each of these results and give reasons for your decision.

Number	Patient's red cells reacted with:				Patient's plasma reacted with:			
	Anti-A	Anti-B	Anti-A,B	Anti-A_1	A_1 RBCs	A_2 RBCs	B RBCs	O RBCs
1	0	0	0	0	3	3	3	0
2	4	0	4	4	0	0	3	0
3	4	4	4	2	0	0	0	0
4	0	3	3	0	3	2	0	0
5	4	0	4	0	2	0	4	0
6	0	0	0	0	3	3	3	3
7	3	3	3	0	0	0	0	0
8	0	2	2	0	0	0	0	0
9	2	0	2	0	0	0	2	0
10	4	4	4	0	2	0	0	0

2. Using the phenotype information, provide possible genotype options for the ten phenotype results obtained.

SECTION 4

THE Rh BLOOD GROUP SYSTEM

The Rh system was originally described in 1939, being erroneously termed the Rhesus system by some US workers due to the fact that much of the early work was performed using antibodies produced in animals (as a result of being injected with rhesus monkey red cells). These antibodies were shown to react with a human red cell antigen (which is now known to be LW) and gave reactions similar to human produced immune antibodies. The human blood group system is now correctly termed Rh (not Rhesus!).

Rh GENES AND ANTIGENS

The Rh gene locus is located on chromosome number 1. DNA studies have shown that there are two Rh genes, *D* and *CE* at this locus. The *D* gene is responsible for the production of the molecule that carries the D antigen and the *CE* gene produces the molecule that contains the antigen combinations ce, Ce, cE or CE dependent upon the gene present. An Rh D negative individual lacks the *D* gene, and D protein, but has the *CE* gene and the CE protein. The D and CE carrier molecules are large proteins that loop through the red cell membrane six times. Each consists of 417 amino acids with very little difference in the amino acid residue sequence.

Rh D negative people do not appear to have any red cell membrane dysfunction that might be expected as a result of the absence of such a major red cell protein. The absence of the D protein also provides an explanation as to why the D antigen appears to be so immunogenic to D negative people (in being able to readily stimulate the production of anti-D). The absence of the *D* gene is by convention identified by the letter 'd' although no allelic status or gene product should be inferred.

Although the *D* and *CE* locus genes each produce a separate protein, they are inserted into the red cell membrane next to each other, thereby producing a complex of antigens. The presence or absence of the *D* gene, together with one of the four *CE* gene options results in eight possible gene or haplotype combinations. Therefore a person may produce various combinations of these antigens dependant upon which haplotypes they have inherited.

Rh Nomenclature

CE GENE	D GENE	
	D	*d*
Ce	*CDe*	*Cde*
cE	*cDE*	*cdE*
ce	*cDe*	*cde*
CE	*CDE*	*CdE*

Each of the eight haplotype gene complexes are possible, each of which has been given a 'shorthand' notation. The use of 'R' indicates the presence of the *D* gene, whereas the use of 'r' indicates its absence (i.e. 'd'). These are identified in the following table:

D GENE *	CE GENE	HAPLOTYPE GENE COMPLEX	'SHORTHAND' NOMENCLATURE
D	*Ce*	*CDe*	R_1
D	*cE*	*cDE*	R_2
D	*ce*	*cDe*	R_o
D	*CE*	*CDE*	R_z
d	*ce*	*cde*	r
d	*Ce*	*Cde*	r'
d	*cE*	*cdE*	r''
d	*CE*	*CdE*	r^y

* The absence of the D gene is indicated in this table by a *d* symbol. It is recognised that no *d* gene exists and as such, the letter *d* is used to represent the absence of *D*.

A haplotype (the presence or absence of *D* together with one of the four *CE* gene options) is inherited from each parent. The genotype of an individual is therefore composed of the combination of any two of the eight possible haplotypes, one from each parent. A total of 32 genotype combinations are therefore theoretically possible, though some of these are extremely rare (see below). The genotype may be written as either haplotype combinations or in the shorthand notation, for example:

cde / cde   or   rr

CDe / cde   or R_1r

cDE / cdE   or R_2r''

The fact that Rh genes segregate (in inheritance) as haplotypes can be illustrated by the possible offspring of selected matings, e.g. of the genotypes R_1R_2 x $r'r$

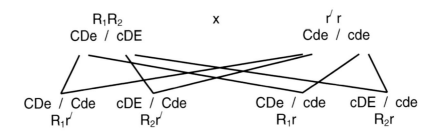

Many rare Rh variant genes have also been described, which are believed to occur due to a variety of genetic causes (e.g. mutation, crossing-over, gene conversion, etc.). These genes have been shown to result in the production of Rh antigens that give variable results with normal Rh antisera.

Rh FREQUENCIES

The frequencies of the eight possible Rh haplotype gene combinations vary within a given population, and between different populations. As a result, the frequency of individual genotypes vary, making some genotypes relatively common (e.g. R_1R_1) whilst others are very rare (e.g. $r'r''$).

The 'commonest' Rh types

Rh TYPE	PHENOTYPE RESULTS WITH :					PERCENTAGE FREQUENCY *
	Anti-D	Anti-C	Anti-c	Anti-E	Anti-e	
R_1R_1	4	4	0	0	4	18
R_2R_2	4	0	4	4	0	3
R_1R_2	4	4	4	4	4	13
R_1r	4	4	4	0	4	35
R_2r	4	0	4	4	4	12
R_o	4	0	4	0	4	2
rr	0	0	4	0	4	15
$r'r$	0	4	4	0	4	0.4
$r''r$	0	0	4	4	4	0.8
$r'r'$	0	4	0	0	4	<0.1
$r''r''$	0	0	4	4	0	<0.1
$r'r''$	0	4	4	4	4	<0.1

* Approximate frequency in UK blood donors (frequencies vary in different ethnic groups).
Notes: R_z and r^y are not included due to their rarity.
R_o is more common in Black populations (i.e. frequency ~ 50%).
The genotype rr is rare in Chinese (i.e. frequency ~ 0.3%).
The term R_o is used in this table to represent the phenotypically indistinguishable R_oR_o and R_or (the frequency of which varies between Black and White populations).

Rh ANTIGENS

The Rh antigens, coded for by the Rh genes, are known to be non-glycosylated non-phosphorylated trans-membrane proteins. There is known to be a high degree of homology between the D and CE proteins, with cDNA studies showing them each to consist of 417 amino acids. The D protein spans the red cell membrane 12 times, therefore providing six extracellular domains, arranged in a complex circle-like formation.

A simplified two-dimensional representation of the D polypeptide

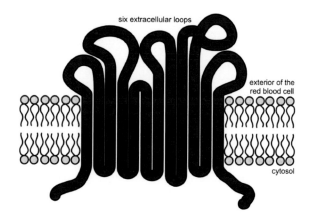

Sequence analysis of different CE proteins has shown that the C and c specificities differ by only 4 amino acids, whilst the E and e specificities differ by a single amino acid substitution within the total protein. The Rh proteins within the red cell membrane have a trans-membrane transport role. The D and CE proteins appear to have a similar if not identical function.

The D antigen

The D antigen is characterised by being very antigenic (it gives very strong reactions with its antibody), is strongly immunogenic (in being able to stimulate antibody production) and is the most clinically significant of the Rh antigens, especially with regard to Haemolytic Disease of the Fetus/Newborn (HDFN). The D antigen, together with its antibody, is second only to the ABO blood group system antigens in clinical importance.

Immunisation by the D antigen is more likely to result in immune antibody stimulation than any other red cell antigen. Approximately 60% of D- people transfused with one or more units of D+ red cells will produce anti-D. Of the non-Rh antigens, the K antigen of the Kell blood group system is the next most immunogenic. By comparison only approximately 10% of K- people will develop anti-K following a single transfusion of K+ red cells. Approximately one third of all non-Rh red cell immune antibodies are anti-K. An immunogenicity comparison of this kind however must also take into account the respective antigen frequencies seen in the random population. The D+ antigen frequency of approximately 85% ensures that D- people would frequently be randomly immunised by D+ blood. By comparison, the K+ antigen frequency of approximately 10% reduces the likelihood of a K- person being randomly immunised by a K+ transfusion.

The Rh antigens are generally well developed at birth, the D antigen having been identified on red cells very early in fetal life (at 38 days). Molecular genetic testing offers the opportunity of D genotyping small quantities of genomic DNA, permitting D typing of fetal cells obtained either by chorionic-villus biopsy or amniocentesis or more usually from the minute amounts of fetal DNA that can be found in the maternal plasma. This is important for assessing the D antigen status of the fetus of a woman who has a pre-formed high titre anti-D and whose D+ partner is potentially heterozygote (*Dd*), i.e. to assess if the fetus is D+ and therefore capable of suffering from HDFN.

Studies have indicated that the D antigen site distribution on the red cell membrane is non-random, which is believed to be the reason why IgG anti-D sera are unable to activate complement *in vitro* and *in vivo*.

The number of D antigen sites per red cell varies widely, dependant upon the Rh phenotype/genotype. The values obtained using radio-labelled anti-D can be summarised as follows:

RED CELL GENOTYPE		D ANTIGEN SITE NUMBERS PER RED CELL (approximate)
CDe / cde	R_1r	10,000 - 15,000
CDe / CDe	R_1R_1	15,000 - 20,000
cDE / cDE	R_2R_2	16,000 - 33,000
-D- / -D-	CE deletion	111,000 - 202,000

Rh D exhibits 'dosage effects', i.e. more antigen is produced per red cell by the *D* homozygote (e.g. CDe/CDe) than the *D* heterozygote (e.g. CDe/cde). In addition, there is a quantitative variation in D antigen expression that is reflected at a practical level by the variable reactivity of certain Rh phenotypes with some anti-D reagents, the strongest D reacting red cell being -D-/-D-, followed by R_2R_2 and R_1R_1 phenotypes. There is less D antigen expression detected when Ce is present compared with cE, i.e. R_1r reacts weaker than R_2r with anti-D. Agglutination titres and flow cytometry have identified a decreasing D reactivity between red cell phenotypes to be cDE/cDE > CDe/cDE > CDe/CDe > cDE/cde > CDe/cde.

WEAK D (previously called D^u)

The term D^u has been replaced with the more accurate term 'weak D'. A 'weak D' group results from the presence of fewer D antigen sites per red cell compared to normal D antigen expression, a quantitative effect, and is an inherited characteristic. Molecular studies have shown that there are a number of different changes to the D gene that give rise to changes in the D carrier molecule that are within the red cell and not on the outside of the cell (i.e. non-exofacial). These changes give rise to a weakened D antigen expression and have been designated as *weak D type 1*, *weak D type 2*, etc.

Different weak D phenotypes may exhibit a range of D antigenic expression and may vary with the type and origin of the anti-D reagents used. Most monoclonal anti-D reagents give a normal strength reaction with many examples of weak D when compared with some polyclonal anti-D sera.

Where there is a discrepancy in the D typing results using the two routine anti-D typing reagents, the patient should be treated as D negative and given D negative red cells until the problem is resolved. Although there appears to be no conclusive evidence that the weak D type is responsible for the primary stimulation of anti-D, blood donors are tested by sensitive methods with two examples of potent anti-D reagents to detect weak D antigen expression. If identified as a weak D type, the donor (and donation) is called Rh D positive (see Section 13: Blood Donation Testing).

It is less important to detect weak D types in recipients, since the consequences of grouping a weak D recipient as D negative will result in that person (who is actually D positive), receiving D negative blood without any ill effects. Individuals who have weak D antigen expression are incapable of forming anti-D and therefore giving them D positive red cells will also result in no ill effects. As such, the testing of D negative patient's samples with AHG reactive IgG anti-D ("a D^u test") to identify if the person is actually a weak D type is not recommended.

D VARIANTS

There have been described a very small number of individuals whose red cells express a variant D protein resulting from changes in their inherited D gene. These result in a small change to the amino acid sequence in the part of the D carrier molecule that is on the outside of the red cell, or exofacial. As these red cells often give variable reactions with anti-D reagents they are frequently referred to as 'partial D' types. Based on this reactivity, D variants have been categorised into a number of different categories, e.g. II, IIIa, IIIb, IIIc, IVa, IVb, Va, Vb, VI and VII. The molecular basis for these categories is known but as additional minor variations continue to be described it is increasingly difficult to put them all into categories that were based purely on serological findings.

Individuals with these rare types, especially those termed D category VI, which has the least amount of D antigen of the variant D types are capable of making anti-D if transfused with D positive blood, i.e. they make an antibody to the D antigen portion which they lack. Therefore although anti-D reagents are selected for blood donor testing which are capable of detecting these variant D antigens, the antisera used for the grouping of patient's red cells should be selected to not detect category VI types. These people will then be classified as Rh D negative and therefore they will be transfused only with D negative blood.

Cc AND Ee ANTIGENS

The C / c and E / e antigens have the following UK antigen frequencies:

ANTIGEN	APPROXIMATE ANTIGEN FREQUENCY (UK)
C	70%
C	81%
E	30%
E	98%

These Rh antigens are less immunogenic than D. The C antigen stimulates the production of anti-C in only approximately 2% of C negative people after a single transfusion event. These antigens exhibit some dosage effects between homozygotes and heterozygotes (dependent upon the grouping sera used). Like the D antigen, a number of variants have been described, most of which are rare in Whites.

C^w

Although originally believed to be produced by an allele of *C* and *c* genes, C^w is allelic to a high incidence antigen MAR. C^w is a relatively low frequency antigen occurring in only approximately 3% of the UK population. C^w positive red cells are almost always C+, but the antigen associated with C^w is weaker than normal C. C^w is frequently associated with the CDe gene complex. Anti-C^w is not an uncommon antibody, frequently appearing to be 'naturally occurring' and may be clinically significant in causing (mild) HDFN.

G AND ANTI-G

The Rh C and D proteins share the same amino-acid sequence from position 50 to 103. Anti-G recognises a serine amino acid at position 103, which is common to both the C and D proteins. As a result, red cells which are either C+ or D+ are also G+. Only as a great rarity have red cells been found which are either C-D- but G+ (called r^G), or C+ and/or D+ but G negative. Red cells that are weak D (and C-) react weakly with anti-G. Therefore, many anti-C+D sera have an additional anti-G component, formed due to the fact that all C+ and/or D+ red cells, which would be capable of stimulating the formation of such antibodies, are also G positive. Anti-G can be separated by adsorption-elution experiments from sera containing anti-C+D. As a result, it is obvious that anti-G will appear to be an anti-C+D in routine antibody identification studies. Some examples of anti-G may give weaker reactions against ccDEE phenotype red cells compared with CCDee phenotype red cells. This is untypical of anti-C+D.

There have been a small number of cases described where cde/cde (rr) women have produced apparent anti-C+D antibodies when their partners are D+C- (cDE or cDe) or D-C+ (Cde or CdE), or when they have delivered Cde/cde (r'r) children. These cases can be explained by the fact that the apparent anti-C+D specificities are actually anti-G or anti-C+G.

The strong immunogenicity of the G antigen may also explain why the C antigen is such an ineffective immunising agent in cDE/cde people compared with cde/cde people. In such situations, the immunising C+G+ red cells may be seen as 'less foreign' to a C-G+ (cDE/cde) person than to a C-G- (cde/cde) person. Therefore, an anti-C produced by a cDE/cde (R_2r) person is 'pure' (no possible anti-G component)

DELETIONS AND SUPPRESSIONS OF Rh

A variety of gene deletions and suppressions involving various parts of the Rh complex have been described (e.g. -D-/-D-, Rh_{null}, cD-/cD-, C^wD-, etc.), in which some or all of the expected Rh antigens are missing from the red cell membrane. These are mainly the result of gene deletions, all of which are rare. There is a high consanguinity rate among the parents of these phenotype people.

-D- types

The genetic background of the -D- phenotype is heterogeneous. Molecular genetic studies have identified the cause to be a deletion of the *CE* gene, although suppression of a normal *CE* gene is also a possibility. The red cells of -D- phenotype people therefore only express D and G antigens. The *-D-* gene complex is very rare with some examples having been described in paternity cases due to apparent exclusion of parentage. The parents of -D- people appear to be 'apparent homozygotes', i.e.

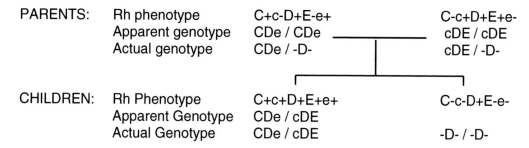

PARENTS:	Rh phenotype	C+c-D+E-e+		C-c+D+E+e-
	Apparent genotype	CDe / CDe		cDE / cDE
	Actual genotype	CDe / -D-		cDE / -D-

CHILDREN:	Rh Phenotype	C+c+D+E+e+		C-c-D+E-e-
	Apparent Genotype	CDe / cDE		
	Actual Genotype	CDe / cDE		-D- / -D-

The red cells of people homozygous (and heterozygous) for -D- express more D antigen than normal D+ (either *DD* or *Dd*) red cells. This increased number of D antigen sites per red cell is the reason why polyclonal IgG anti-D sera can directly agglutinate -D- red cells in a saline medium.

People who are homozygous -D- types are readily immunised by common Rh phenotype red cells via either pregnancy and/or transfusion, to produce an antibody (i.e. anti-Hr_o or anti-RH17), which is capable of reacting with all red cells except other Rh deletion and Rh_{null} red cell types. This is a clinically significant 37^oC reacting antibody, capable of causing severe, often fatal, HDFN. The presence of this antibody is normally the reason why these very rare phenotype people are identified in the first place. Because of the presence of this antibody, all subsequent transfusions must only be with -D- (or Rh_{null}) red cells.

Rh deficiency syndrome (Rh_{null} phenotype)

The Rh_{null} phenotype is the absence of normal expression of all Rh antigens, i.e. it gives a Rh phenotype result of C-c-D-E-e-. The absence of the Rh proteins results in a defective red cell membrane producing a shortened red cell survival and (usually) a compensated clinical anaemia ("Rh_{null} disease"). This is a very rare condition and has been demonstrated to be due to two different genetic backgrounds.

The 'amorphic' type of Rh_{null} is caused by the presence of silent alleles at the Rh locus (i.e. written ---/---). The parents and children of amorphic Rh_{null} people are heterozygous for the silent gene. Initial phenotype testing identifies the parents of Rh_{null} people to be 'apparent homozygotes', however their red cells give heterozygous reactions in dosage studies with selected Rh antisera indicating them to be in fact heterozygote for the silent gene. The presence in a family of the amorphic gene (---) may cause apparent Rh inheritance problems. It is inherited in an identical manner to the -D- haplotype (see above).

An example of amorphic type Rh_{null} inheritance

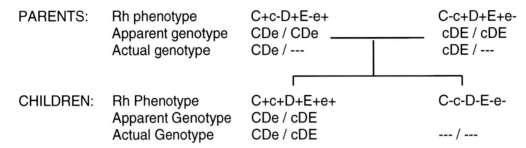

PARENTS:	Rh phenotype	C+c-D+E-e+		C-c+D+E+e-
	Apparent genotype	CDe / CDe		cDE / cDE
	Actual genotype	CDe / ---		cDE / ---

CHILDREN:	Rh Phenotype	C+c+D+E+e+	C-c-D-E-e-
	Apparent Genotype	CDe / cDE	
	Actual Genotype	CDe / cDE	--- / ---

The 'regulator' type Rh_{null} is very rare and results from the homozygote inheritance of an inactivating mutation of the *RHAG* gene, present on chromosome 6 (the Rh gene is on chromosome 1 and *RhAG* is therefore not linked to the Rh gene). Note: the 'regulator' gene was originally called $X^{o}r$. The presence of normal RhAG (Rh associated glycoprotein) is a requirement for the normal expression of red cell Rh antigens; an abnormality in RhAG results in abnormal Rh antigen expression, even in the presence of normal *RHD* and *RHCE* genes. The parents and offspring of regulator type Rh_{null} are heterozygous for the abnormal *RhAG* gene and therefore have normal Rh antigen expression.

Example of regulator type Rh_{null} inheritance

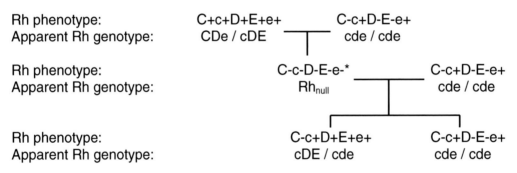

| Rh phenotype: | C+c+D+E+e+ | C-c+D-E-e+ |
| Apparent Rh genotype: | CDe / cDE | cde / cde |

| Rh phenotype: | C-c-D-E-e-* | C-c+D-E-e+ |
| Apparent Rh genotype: | Rh_{null} | cde / cde |

| Rh phenotype: | C-c+D+E+e+ | C-c+D-E-e+ |
| Apparent Rh genotype: | cDE / cde | cde / cde |

* The children of this person have inherited the haplotypes cDE and cde illustrating this person to be Rh genotype R_2r though the Rh genes are not expressed due to having inherited two abnormal *RHAG* genes (i.e. the parents of this person are both heterozygous for an abnormal *RHAG* gene).

Immunisation, as a result of transfusion and/or pregnancy, frequently stimulates Rh_{null} people to produce an antibody that reacts equally well with all red cell phenotypes, except other Rh_{null} types. This antibody is known as anti-Rh29 or anti-'total Rh' (a high frequency antigen present on all red cells other than Rh_{null}).

Rh ANTIBODIES

The vast majority of Rh antibodies produced by patients are IgG, though some (especially examples of anti-C) may have a strong IgM component. Rh antibodies are immune and react optimally at 37°C, though a number of 'naturally occurring' Rh antibodies (anti-E, anti-C^w and anti-c) have been described. Most react well by both enzyme and anti-human globulin (AHG) techniques. Some examples react only by enzyme techniques ("enzyme only antibodies"), which are not clinically significant in transfusion. Rh antibodies are clinically significant in being able to cause transfusion reactions (including delayed transfusion reactions) and HDFN. Although Rh antibodies do not activate complement they are still capable of causing the destruction of incompatible red cells *in vivo* since the IgG antibody coated red cells are detected by macrophages in the spleen and removed from the circulation. Some Rh antibodies are produced as mixtures, either as mixtures of different Rh antibody specificities (e.g. anti-C+D, anti-C+D+E, anti-c+E, etc.) or together with antibodies to other non-Rh antigens (e.g. anti-D+K, anti-D+E+Fy^a, etc.).

Anti-D

This antibody specificity may be produced by D negative women as a result of fetal red cell stimulation occurring from feto-maternal haemorrhage during pregnancy and/or at delivery. It is infrequently produced as a result of transfusion due to the routine use of D negative blood for D negative recipients. The antibody is capable of showing dosage effects. Anti-D often occurs together with other Rh and non-Rh antibody specificities. Anti-D is an extremely clinically important antibody specificity in both transfusion and especially HDFN.

Anti-c

This antibody is usually produced in R_1R_1 people, since the frequency of the other potential genotype producers (R_1r', $r'r$, etc.) are rare. It may be found as either a single antibody specificity or together with anti-E (when immunised with R_1R_2, R_2R_2 or R_2r red cells) and is usually a mixture of IgG+IgM. Anti-c is clinically the most important of the Rh antibody specificities after anti-D and is capable of causing severe HDFN.

Anti-C

Pure anti-C is a rare antibody and is more commonly produced in combination with anti-D (by cde/cde genotype pregnant women) or together with anti-e (by R_2R_2 genotype people immunised with C+e+ blood). Anti-C is usually a combination of IgG+IgM and may exhibit dosage effects. Anti-C seldom causes HDFN and if it does, the disease is usually mild.

Anti-E

Pure anti-E occurs more frequently than pure anti-C, sometimes as an apparently 'naturally occurring' antibody. Some examples may react only by enzyme techniques ("enzyme-only"), in which case they are considered to be clinically insignificant in transfusion. When produced by R_1R_1 people in response to immunisation by R_2r (or R_2R_2) phenotype red cells, it may be produced together with anti-c. Some examples may give variable reactions by LISS-IAT, sensitive enzyme or gel techniques. Anti-E seldom causes HDFN and if it does, the disease is usually mild.

Anti-e

This is a very rare alloantibody due to the antigen being a weak immunogen and also due to the rarity of Rh genotypes (E+e-) that are able to produce the antibody. If produced, the antibody is frequently weak and usually reacts best by enzyme techniques. Anti-e seldom causes HDFN and if it does, the disease is invariably mild. Apparent auto-anti-e is not an uncommon antibody.

Rh GROUPING (PHENOTYPING)

Rh phenotyping is performed by grouping the red cell sample using two examples of each specific anti-Rh reagent (anti-D, anti-C, anti-E, anti-c and anti-e). The detected Rh antigen combination is known as the red cell phenotype. For example:

REACTIONS WITH ANTISERA:					ANTIGENS PRESENT / RED CELL PHENOTYPE
ANTI-C	ANTI-D	ANTI-E	ANTI-c	ANTI-e	
Pos	Pos	Neg	Pos	Pos	CcDe
Neg	Pos	Pos	Pos	Pos	cDEe

It is impossible to determine accurately the Rh genotype of an individual from the Rh phenotype (grouping results) obtained, but a possible genotype may be deduced based on known haplotype frequencies (calculated from family studies and population data). However, since the incidence of the different haplotypes varies between races, the estimation of the 'probable genotype' must be treated with caution.

For example:

Rh PHENOTYPE	POSSIBLE GENOTYPES		ACTUAL % FREQUENCY OF GENOTYPE (Whites)
CcDe	CDe / cde	R_1r	35% *
	CDe / cDe	R_1R_0	2%
	cDe / Cde	R_0r'	<0.1%
cDEe	cDE / cde	R_2r	12% *
	cDE / cDe	R_2R_0	0.7%
	cDe / cdE	R_0r''	<0.1%

* These would therefore be the "most probable" genotypes calculated from the phenotype results obtained.

The phenotype results cannot indicate if a red cell sample is homozygous (*DD*) or heterozygous (*Dd*) for the *D* gene, since there is no *d* gene antigenic product. Therefore, although it is not always possible to deduce the Rh genotype from the phenotype results obtained, knowledge of the haplotype frequencies allows the determination of the 'most probable genotype'. It is important also to note that very rare Rh gene complexes, such as for example cD-, -D- as well as --- (where the '-' symbol indicates the absence of a gene), will affect phenotype result frequencies and possible genotype option calculations.

Testing of blood donors

All new donor blood samples are routinely tested with two examples of monoclonal anti-D reagents. Only those found to be negative with both antisera are classified as Rh D negative (see also weak D types, above). Donations are further tested by the blood services in the UK to identify their Rh phenotype and K group (see Section 13: Blood Donation Testing).

Testing of transfusion recipients (patients)

Patients should be tested in duplicate using monoclonal anti-D grouping reagent (i.e. using the same reagent twice or two different reagents). The two tests may involve antibody derived from the same or different clones and should be controlled by the use of D+ and D- red cell samples. If found to be D negative the patient should be transfused with Rh D negative blood only; if found to be D positive the patient should be transfused with Rh D positive blood. This policy avoids the risk of a D negative person being transfused with the D antigen and therefore the possible stimulation of anti-D by the patient is prevented, whilst in addition, conserving the Rh D negative blood stock. It is however also possible for certain D negative patients (i.e. males) to receive D positive blood in an emergency if the amount of blood required for the patient is large (e.g. for a liver transplant) and the available D negative blood stock is low.

This system of D grouping does not however avoid a recipient receiving blood containing an antigen that they lack and therefore potentially stimulating the production of an antibody (or antibodies). This policy is based on the knowledge that the red cell antigens other than D are weaker immunogens and only infrequently stimulates antibody production. However, for patients who need to be supported during their life time by repeated transfusions, blood should be selected which is Rh and K phenotype compatible with the patient, so as to prevent antibodies to these antigens being formed. Although less immunogenic than D, this illustrates the higher immunogenicity potential of Rh and K antigens in comparison to those of the other blood group systems.

All Rh antibodies are capable of causing severe transfusion reactions, therefore the laboratory testing of blood donors and transfusion recipients is designed to:
a. Prevent the stimulation of anti-D antibodies as a result of transfusion by ensuring that D negative individuals are transfused with D negative red cells.
b. Detect the presence of any Rh antibodies in the recipient's serum/plasma and avoid the transfusion of antigen positive red cells by the provision of antigen negative and cross-match compatible blood.

For information regarding the clinical significance of Rh in causing HDFN, see Section 11: Haemolytic disease of the Fetus/Newborn.

ABO AND RhD BLOOD GROUP INCIDENCE

Approximately 80-90% of European and North American White people (85% in the UK), 95% of Black Africans and almost 100% of Chinese and Japanese peoples have the D red cell antigen, i.e. are D+. In the UK blood donor population, this equates to the following frequencies when combined with individual ABO groups:

GROUP	APPROXIMATE UK FREQUENCY	PERCENTAGE Rh D POSITIVE (85%)	PERCENTAGE Rh D NEGATIVE (15%)
A	43%	36.6%	6.5%
B	9%	7.6%	1.4%
O	45%	38.25%	6.75%
AB	3%	2.5%	0.5%

QUESTIONS - SECTION 4

1. What percentage of the UK population is D positive and D negative?

2. Why is it not necessary to test patient samples for weak D (D^u) antigen?

3. State which CcDEe antigens are represented by the following haplotypes:

   a. R_1
   b. R_2
   c. r
   d. r'
   e. r''
   f. R_o.

4. Why is the D antigen believed to be so strongly immunogenic?

5. Can 'weak D' and 'variant D' types produce anti-D?

6. What approximate percentage of the UK population are O Rh D negative, O Rh D positive, A Rh D negative and A Rh D positive?

7. Which of the Rh antibodies are capable of causing destruction of incompatible red cells?

8. What genotype are the fetal D positive red cells that stimulate a D negative woman to produce anti-D?

9. What are the phenotype and most probable genotypes from the following Rh blood grouping results?

	Results obtained with:				
	Anti-D	Anti-C	Anti-c	Anti-E	Anti-e
Sample A	4	4	4	4	4
Sample B	0	0	4	4	4
Sample C	4	4	0	0	4
Sample D	4	0	4	4	4
Sample E	0	4	4	0	4

10. Which are the Rh antibodies most likely to cause Haemolytic Disease of the Fetus/Newborn?

ASSIGNMENT

Using the data collected from your Blood Bank records, calculate the frequencies of the ABO and Rh D blood groups (e.g. as A Rh D positive, B Rh D negative, etc.) of both the patients and donations cross-matched.

Is there a significant difference between them, and if so, can you suggest why?

ABO/Rh DATA INTERPRETATION - SECTIONS 3 AND 4

The following table represents the ABO and Rh D blood grouping results from testing 12 different patients' blood samples. All reagents and techniques have been checked and are working correctly (i.e. the results depicted are not the result of clerical or technical error). All control results are as expected. Interpret the results so as to provide the ABO and Rh D blood groups (phenotypes) for each patient and comment on any unusual finding.

No	ANTI-			ANTI-		RC	RED CELLS			
	A	B	A,B	D(1)	D(2)		A₁	A₂	B	O
1	4	0	4	0	0	0	0	0	3	0
2	0	4	4	4	4	0	4	3	0	0
3	0	0	0	1	1	0	4	3	4	0
4	4	0	4	0	0	0	2	0	4	0
5	0	0	0	0	0	0	4	4	4	4
6	4	4	4	4	4	0	0	0	0	0
7	2mf	0	2mf	4	4	0	0	0	3	0
8	0	4	4	2	0	0	2	2	0	0
9	2	4	4	0	0	0	2	0	0	0
10	4	0	4	4	3	0	0	1	4	3
11	0	4	4	0	0	0	1	1	0	0
12	0	0	0	0	0	0	0	0	0	0

RC: Reagent control (see Section 5: Basic Serological Techniques and Controls)
mf: Mixed field result

For those readers who are unfamiliar with the grading system used in the above chart, they are referred to the chart 'Standardised grading system for the recording of agglutination' within Section 5.

SECTION 5

BASIC SEROLOGICAL TECHNIQUES AND CONTROLS

NOTE:
The authors recognise that an increasing number of pathology laboratories employ automated technologies for performing routine blood grouping and antibody detection, with a concomitant reduction in the routine use of manual techniques. Although this is recognised to be the case, the authors believe that teaching the theory as well and the practical aspects of manual techniques will illustrate their underlying principles as well as methodologies. It is important that the student understands 'what is going on'. There will no doubt be a time, in the possibly not too distant future, when all laboratories are completely automated. Until that time, and whilst some laboratories use at least a limited degree of manual techniques, this and the following chapter will continue to be included in this book.

There are a number of different manual techniques that continue to be used routinely within blood transfusion laboratories. Those described below are examples of the basic techniques employed, which may vary in methodology from one laboratory to another. Other technique options may be equally valid.

SALINE / DIRECT AGGLUTINATION TECHNIQUE

In a suitable tube (i.e. precipitin or 75x12mm) or microplate well, add the following:

- 1 volume of serum/plasma, i.e. one drop from a (plastic) Pasteur pipette or an equivalent volume (~30µl) from an automatic pipette
- 1 drop (equivalent volume) of a 2-3% red blood cell suspension in phosphate buffered saline
- Mix the contents of the tube by gently shaking (for microplates, mix by agitation, preferably on a mixer)

The tube can then be either centrifuged immediately (the "immediate spin" technique), or incubated at an appropriate temperature for 10-30 minutes, before centrifugation.

Reading the results
Hold the tube over a light source and look for haemolysis, then tip and role the tube gently a few times to dislodge the red cell button and look for agglutination.

Recording the results
Positive results must be graded according to the strength of agglutination observed, e.g. in decreasing order of strength as: ++++, +++, ++ and + though an equivalent numerical system for identifying the strength of agglutination of 4, 3, 2, and 1 is increasingly being used. Un-agglutinated red cells should be recorded as neg or "0". If the cells are haemolysed, record as L (lysis). For the definition of these reactions refer to the table later in this section.

TWO-STAGE (PRE-MODIFICATION) PAPAIN TECHNIQUE

Stage One:
Enzyme modification of red cells:
- Dilute the stock of 1% papain 1 in 10 in saline (this may vary from batch to batch)
- To one drop of packed washed red cells add 4 drops of diluted papain solution
- Mix well
- Incubate at 37°C in a water bath for 12 minutes (or as per package insert)
- Wash the red cells twice in saline
- Re-suspend the red cells to 2-3% in saline. These red cells can be used for up to 24 hours

Stage Two:
Proceed as with the direct agglutination technique, but incubate a 37°C for 20 minutes.

Controls
Positive: Weak anti-D with D positive (OR$_1$r) red cells.
Negative: AB serum with D positive (OR$_1$r) red cells.

Notes
Enzyme techniques are not usually used for pre-transfusion antibody screening of patients but are recommended when performing antibody identification panels to determine the specificity of an antibody.

Enzyme techniques may be prone to 'non-specific' positive results and for producing positive results that are not confirmed by other techniques, e.g. IAT. These positive results are produced due to the effects of the enzyme treatment on red cell membrane proteins. By removing some protein, enzyme treatment exposes previously hidden structures enabling them to react with immunoglobulins present in the patient's serum/plasma, resulting in 'non-specific' positive results. Other red cell antigens become more exposed (accessible to antibody reaction) following enzyme treatment, this is especially true for Rh antigens. As a result, some examples of weakly reacting antibody specificities may react with enzyme treated red cells, but not with non-enzyme treated examples of the same red cells, these are therefore known as "enzyme only antibodies". These antibodies are not clinically significant in transfusion, i.e. if antigen positive red cells are transfused in the presence of these antibodies their survival is not compromised. Similarly, there is no evidence to support the concept that the titre of an 'enzyme only' antibody is increased or its reactivity broadened, following the transfusion of antigen positive red cells to patients with enzyme only reactive antibodies.

LOW IONIC STRENGTH SALINE (LISS) INDIRECT ANTIGLOBULIN TEST (IAT).
NOTE : See also Section 6: The Anti-Human Globulin Test.

Preparation of red cells
Wash the red cells twice in saline and then once in LISS.
Re-suspend the red cells to a 1.5%-2% suspension in LISS.

Indirect antiglobulin tube test
- In a 75x12mm tube place equal volumes of serum/plasma and LISS suspended red cells, i.e. 2 drops of serum and 2 drops of red cells in LISS
- Mix the contents well
- Incubate at 37°C for 15-20 minutes
- Look for haemolysis and/or agglutination - if present the test is positive

- Wash the red cells 3 (or4) times in saline
- Add 2 drops of anti-human globulin (AHG) reagent, mix
- Gently centrifuge the tube
- Read and record the reactions

Negative test control

Add one drop of IgG sensitised red cells, mix and gently centrifuge then read.
Agglutination should now be present. If still negative, the test must be repeated (see Section 6: The Anti-Human Globulin Test).

Note: The above techniques use traditional "liquid phase" tube technology. U-well microplates can be used in place of tubes for saline (direct) techniques and are widely used for ABO and D typing.

MICROCOLUMN TECHNIQUES

Together with microplate technology, 'microcolumn' techniques (involving the use of microcolumns / microtubes containing either glass micro-beads or a matrix of gel (marketed as either DiaMed-ID™ or Ortho BioVue™), are used by most blood transfusion laboratories for routine ABO and D grouping, antibody screening and/or crossmatching procedures.

Both of the available commercial systems consist of 'cards', each holding six microcolumns. With the basic system, the top of each microcolumn is wider to form a 'reaction chamber' where the red cell and serum/plasma mixture is incubated (see illustrations below), with a lower narrower area containing a matrix of either sephadex gel or glass micro-beads. Therefore, when the cards are centrifuged, the matrix traps red cell agglutinates, i.e. on the surface or within the column (indicating a positive result) whereas un-agglutinated cells move through the matrix forming a button at the base of the microcolumn (indicating a negative result).

The 'cards' can also be obtained for use in saline techniques with antisera added to the matrix, such as anti-A, anti-B, anti-D, etc., for red cell grouping. This technology can also be used for anti-human globulin testing (see Section 6: The Anti-Human Globulin Test).

Standardised grading system for the recording of agglutination

Strength of reaction		Description of the red cell reaction observed	Titration score
Graded	Numerical		
++++	5	RBC button remains in one clump or dislodges into a few large clumps	12
+++	4	RBC button dislodges into several large clumps	10
++	3	RBC button dislodges into many medium sized / small clumps	8
+	2	RBC button dislodges into finely granular but definite clumps	5
(+)	1	RBC dislodges into very small clumps that are more distinct if the tube is left on its side to allow the red cells to settle, or viewed microscopically	3
-	0	Negative result	0

The 'titration score' values can be used where a quantitative result is required, for example when comparing antibody titres and/or the avidity of antigen-antibody reactions. The 'numerical' reaction method of recording the strength of a reaction is clearer and is less likely to be misinterpreted than the 'graded' method. Irrespective of which notation is used, it is important that the strength of a reaction is recorded for future reference, and that the test result is not just recorded as 'positive' or 'negative'.

Red cell reactions may be viewed either unaided or with the use of a mirror/lens system (a microscope may also be used for identifying the strength of agglutination in tube techniques).

Additional recorded results

Haemolysis:
Designated by the letter H (haemolysis) or L (lysis) and is often graded as strong, medium and trace.

Mixed Field:
The presence of two populations of cells, one clearly agglutinated (positive) and the other clearly unagglutinated (negative). Designated by the letters 'mf' together with an indication of the strength of agglutination of the positive cell population.

Rouleaux:
Non-specific 'pseudoagglutination' due to high concentrations of serum proteins or dextran in the patient's serum/plasma. This type of pseudoagglutination is characteristic in that the red cells appear as 'stacks of coins', i.e. aligned side to side. Rouleaux presence is designated by the letter R.

Strengths of reaction in microcolumns

The following photographs illustrate increasing strengths of positive reactions occurring in microcolumns, from negative on the left via increasingly positive reactions to a strong positive on the right, i.e. as illustrated by the presence and position of agglutinated red cells within the column.

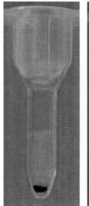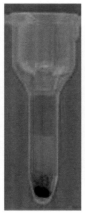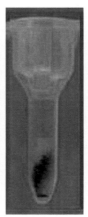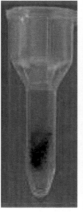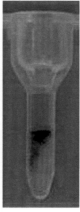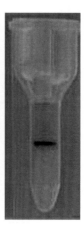

CONTROLS

All blood group serology tests must be adequately controlled. The function of controls is to confirm that the result obtained from the performance of each test is an accurate one. To ensure this, the standard reagents used in each test must be demonstrated to be working correctly. The use of controls also demonstrates that the incubation time and temperature used for the technique are correct. Only by the performance of controls can a positive result be relied upon to be due to a specific reaction and a negative reaction to be accurate and not a "false negative" result.

Although the use of commercial monoclonal reagents has simplified the use of controls (when compared with adsorbed human polyclonal reagents), it has not removed the need for controls since although strong and specific, it is still essential to ensure that the reagents are giving the expected reactions.

Various controls should therefore be routinely used:

Positive control
A positive control is the testing of a specific antiserum with red cells known to express the corresponding antigen, i.e. anti-A with group A red cells. A positive result obtained with this control illustrates that the antisera is working specifically and correctly, and that the technique used has enabled this reaction to have occurred. In antigen grouping using a known specificity antisera against an unknown patient's red cell sample, wherever possible a positive control red cell sample is chosen which has the weakest available expression of the antigen being tested for (e.g. heterozygote expression). The control cell sample is tested against the antisera by the same technique and preferably at the same time as that used to test the unknown (patient's) red cell sample.

Negative control
A negative control illustrates that the reagent antisera used gives specific results. In antigen grouping, this involves the testing of the known specificity antisera with red cell samples that lack the corresponding antigen being tested for, by using the same technique as the test. It is desirable that the negative red cell samples express as many other antigen specificities as possible so that if found negative this control shows the reagent antisera to be specific in its action. If a polyclonal reagent is used, it is usual to choose a red cell sample which expresses the antigens corresponding to the most likely antibody contaminants of other blood group specificities that may be present in the grouping sera. This requirement is of lesser importance and is normally ignored when using a monoclonal reagent, and an antigen negative sample only is used.

Auto (autologous) control
This control is the patient's red cells tested against the patient's serum/plasma sample by the same technique as the test. This control should be negative, since a person cannot normally produce an antibody specificity to which they have the corresponding antigen present on their red cells. A positive auto-control may result from the fact that the patient's red cells or serum/plasma are capable of producing a positive reaction in any test situation, or that the technique conditions are invalid. Irrespective of whether the patient's test result is positive or negative, if the auto control result is positive, the test result cannot be relied upon and the situation must be further investigated.

Note: If an IAT auto test is performed on a patient with a positive DAT it will be positive due to the antibody coating the red cells and not necessarily due to the presence of antibodies in the plasma.

Reagent control

This is sometimes used when (antigen) grouping a red cell sample with a known specificity antiserum. If available, the manufacturer's 'reagent control' (consisting of the diluent or storage medium) must be used as a control for monoclonal reagents, or AB serum (which has been previously tested and found to have no antibodies to any blood group antigen) if a human polyclonal reagent is being used. The reagent control or AB serum is reacted against the test red cell sample by the same technique as used for the grouping sera. If the reagent control or AB serum is positive, the test results cannot be relied upon since it demonstrates that the patient's red cells are non-specifically reactive against any/all sera; therefore the red cells would test non-specifically falsely positive for every antigen specificity.

The necessary controls must be set up at the same time and under the same conditions as the test. Where a large batch of identical tests are performed at the same time, e.g. ABO groups on various samples, only one set of positive and negative controls are required. Test results are invalid unless the correct controls have been used and the results of those tests are as expected. The fact that many grouping reagents used in laboratories are now monoclonal does not negate the need for adequate controls, as these confirm that the reagent is reacting correctly in the technique / situation in which it is being used.

With ABO grouping it is common to control all of the reagents used in a 'checkerboard' manner, whereby each grouping antisera used for the 'cell group' is reacted against each red cell sample used for the 'serum group'. The control of anti-D grouping reagents involves the use of D positive (usually group O R_1r) and D negative (rr) red cell samples.

QUESTIONS - SECTION 5

1. What is an autologous control and what is its purpose?

2. What is a reagent control and what is its purpose?

3. What controls should be used when performing an enzyme technique?

4. Describe the controls required for ABO grouping.

5. Identify the controls required for Rh D grouping.

6. Identify the controls required for Duffy grouping a patient's red cell sample using anti-Fy^a reagent by the AHG technique.

7. What does a positive reaction of a patient's red cells with antibody-free AB serum indicate?

8. What are the two stages of a 'two stage' enzyme technique and what do they achieve?

9. Why are equal volumes of serum/plasma and red cells used in a LISS technique?

10. What methods can be employed to increase the sensitivity of the direct agglutination technique in normal saline?

SECTION 6

THE ANTI-HUMAN GLOBULIN TEST

The anti-human globulin (antiglobulin or AHG) test is also known as the Coombs test, from the surname of one of the discoverers of the technique, i.e. Coombs, Mourant and Race (1945). As the antiglobulin test is the most important technique used in blood bank technology, a complete section is devoted to this test.

PRINCIPLE

After IgG (immunoglobulin) antibody molecules have reacted with their respective antigen on the red cell surface, they are physically too small to bridge the gap between individual red cells in saline. They are unable to accomplish the cross-linking between red cells to produce agglutination and therefore a recognisably positive result. However, IgM antibody molecules are, due to their larger size, able to bridge the gap between red cells in saline to produce agglutination (see Section 2: Antigen-Antibody Reactions). Therefore, unless an alternative test system is used to that involving a saline medium, such as the use of red cell enzyme treatment, the reaction of IgG antibody with its antigen will remain undetected, since agglutination will not occur. The AHG technique is employed to identify the reaction of IgG antibody molecules with their antigen.

The test is performed by the use of a 'sandwich' technique, by the reaction of an antibody to human immunoglobulin, i.e. anti-human globulin or AHG, with antibody sensitised red cells. In this test an antibody to human immunoglobulin, AHG, 'cross-links' the IgG antibody molecules bound to the red cells, producing agglutination (Note: AHG is also capable of reacting with free unbound IgG).

In a tube technique, the red cell and serum/plasma samples are first incubated together (at 37°C) to allow for any antigen-antibody reaction able to take place. After the incubation period, the test should be observed macroscopically for haemolysis and/or agglutination, which if present at this stage identifies that the test must be recorded as positive. A positive result at this stage would indicate the presence of an IgM antibody in the patient's serum/plasma, which is capable of causing direct agglutination or haemolysis in saline). If negative, the red cells (in the tube technique) are then washed in normal phosphate buffered saline to remove any excess serum immunoglobulins, including unbound antibodies. Once the red cells are free of all unbound immunoglobulin, the AHG reagent is added to the washed red cell button. The tests are gently centrifuged and the results read. If an antigen-antibody reaction has occurred, then the anti-human globulin antibody molecules will react with the red cell bound antibody. This results in the cross-linking of the red cells producing agglutinates, which can then be observed. If no antigen-antibody reaction has occurred, then there will be no red cell bound antibody molecules present for the AHG antibodies to bind onto, and therefore no agglutinates will be formed.

If the red cells are not washed free of the contaminating serum prior to the addition of the AHG reagent, the AHG reagent will bind with the excess free immunoglobulin present in all sera, becoming neutralised. The AHG reagent will not therefore be able to produce agglutination, even though there may be blood group antibody bound to the red cells. It is essential therefore that correct procedures, especially for washing the red cells prior to addition of the AHG reagent are closely followed, otherwise false negative results will be obtained. AHG reagent is either produced in an animal immunised with human immunoglobulin or as a monoclonal reagent. The principle of the AHG test is diagrammatically represented at the end of this section.

DIRECT AND INDIRECT TESTS

The prior incubation of red cells and serum/plasma in an AHG technique indicates that the antibody is being allowed to react with the antigen *in vitro* (in the laboratory) and is therefore termed an 'indirect' antiglobulin test (IAT). An indirect test therefore involves two distinct stages. The first stage is where the red cell and serum/plasma samples are incubated together and, following the washing of the test red cell sample, the second stage is the addition of the AHG reagent.

If the red cells from an individual are tested without prior incubation with serum/plasma, this is termed a 'direct' antiglobulin test (or DAT), i.e. the patient's red cell sample is washed in saline and AHG reagent added. This test is used to identify antibody that has reacted with the red cells *in vivo* (in the body). The DAT is performed in various clinical situations, where destruction of red cells by antibody *in vivo* is suspected, such as in Auto-Immune Haemolytic Anaemia (AIHA), a transfusion reaction or Haemolytic Disease of the Fetus/Newborn (HDFN).

SOLID-PHASE RED CELL ADHERENCE (ANTIGLOBULIN TEST) TECHNIQUES

The solid-phase antiglobulin tests (marketed as Immucor Solid-Screen™ or Biotest Solid-Screen™) consists of 'U-well' microplates with either lysed red cell membrane ghosts fixed to the wells as a solid phase, or as microplates which have been 'activated' so that the user can fix their own red cells to the surface of the wells. For use, the test serum/plasma is added to the well(s), together with a low-ionic strength solution and the microplates incubated at 37°C. Because the red cells are fixed to the wells of the microplate, no centrifugation is needed between washes, enabling the saline to be added and then decanted either manually or by the use of an automatic microplate washer.

To visualise positive reactions, indicator red cells coated with AHG reagent are then added. These AHG coated red cells react with (i.e. 'adhere' to) any antibody that has reacted with the red cells coating the wells of the microplate. On centrifugation, positive reactions are seen as a 'carpet' of cells, whereas negative reactions are seen as a button of cells in the bottom of each well. These techniques have been shown to be very sensitive for the detection of IgG antibodies.

MICROCOLUMN (MICROTUBE) TECHNIQUES

Microcolumn technology (see Section 5: Basic Serological Techniques and Controls) also incorporates an AHG test, where the serum/plasma and red cells (in a low-ionic medium) are incubated in the reaction chamber at the top of the 'tube'. The matrix section of 'IAT cards' contains AHG reagent. Therefore after incubation, when the cards are centrifuged, only the red cells and not serum/plasma are heavy enough to enter the matrix and if these are sensitised with IgG antibody they are agglutinated by the AHG reagent and are trapped by the gel or glass-bead matrix. Because only the cells enter the matrix and not the serum/plasma, the free unbound IgG does not mix with the AHG reagent and there is therefore no need to wash the red cells. The technique is therefore much simpler to perform than the tube indirect antiglobulin test (IAT), with fewer possible causes of false positive or negative results. This technology may be performed manually but is frequently employed using an automated testing and reading system.

Even if microcolumn technology is used for AHG testing within your laboratory, it is important to understand the traditional tube technique for IAT and be aware of the problems and/or errors that can occur. It is important, when reading this section, that you compare and contrast the tube and microcolumn AHG techniques.

IgG SENSITISED RED CELL CONTROL

In tube techniques, if the red cell washing procedure is not performed correctly, free unbound serum/plasma immunoglobulin will remain in the red cell test sample. When the AHG reagent is added it binds to the free immunoglobulin, is neutralised and is therefore incapable of reacting with any cell bound immunoglobulin (see above). This is a common cause of false negative reactions in the tube AHG technique, which will be undetectable. However, IgG sensitised control red cells can be used to identify these false negative tests.

IgG sensitised control red cells are prepared by reacting a weak IgG antibody with a selected antigen positive red cell sample (i.e. usually weak anti-D with D positive red cells) and then washing the cells to remove all excess antibody. One drop of these suitably diluted control red cells is added to each negative AHG test. The tube is gently centrifuged and then the result is read again. A true negative AHG test will have the AHG sera still present (i.e. unused) whereas in a 'false negative' the AHG will have been neutralised by the presence of free immunoglobulin. The addition of the control red cells will therefore produce either of the following possibilities:

1. 'The negative test converts to a positive'
   i.e. Agglutination present.
   This indicates a valid negative test result. The IgG sensitised control red cells have been agglutinated by the (unused) AHG reagent present, i.e. free (non-neutralised) AHG reagent is still available in the test and has not been neutralised by free immunoglobulin still present, as a result of incorrect washing.

2. 'The negative test remains negative'
   i.e. No agglutination present.
   This indicates a false negative (invalid) test result. The absence of available AHG reagent in the test able to agglutinate the IgG sensitised control cells must therefore be due to the fact that the AHG reagent has been neutralised by free immunoglobulin, present as a result of an incorrect wash procedure. In this situation, e.g. where the test fails to "convert", the complete procedure must be repeated for the particular test.

THE ROLE OF COMPLEMENT IN AHG TESTING

Complement consists of a group of nine major proteins found in the serum, which are activated by antigen-antibody reactions (see Section 2: Antibody mediated red cell destruction). Under the correct conditions *in vitro*, some antibody molecules, which bind to red cell antigens, are capable of causing the activation and binding to the red cell membrane of the first component of complement (C1). This results in the binding to the red cell of a large number of C3 complement molecules (an example of reaction amplification).

Certain AHG reagents are produced which contain not only anti-human immunoglobulin (IgG) antibodies, but also anti-human complement antibodies (usually anti-C3). Therefore this AHG reagent will 'cross-link' both IgG and complement components if they are both bound to the red cells, making the test more sensitive (by providing a stronger result). The AHG reagents that are produced to contain a mixture of anti-IgG and anti-C3 specificities are called "broad spectrum". Specific anti-IgG and anti-complement AHG reagents are also available. This concept has been used primarily as a means of detecting weak (low titre) antibodies. It is however necessary for a large number of IgG antibodies to be bound per red cell before C1 and therefore C3 are activated. This number of IgG antibodies per red cell is likely to be detected by a good anti-IgG AHG component anyway.

The presence of anticoagulant (EDTA or citrate) in plasma inhibits the complement component C1 and therefore no further complement components are able to be activated, irrespective of the capability of the antigen-antibody reaction to do so. As such, no complement can be bound to the red cells if a plasma sample is used and therefore the anti-C3 present in a 'broad spectrum' AHG reagent is of no use. This fact should be recognised when choosing to use either serum (clotted) or plasma (anticoagulated) samples for blood group serology techniques. Validation of technique and reagent(s) is essential in these situations.

CELL WASHERS - QUALITY CONTROL

Automatic and semi-automatic cell washer machines are commonly used to wash red cell suspensions during the tube AHG procedure. To ensure that a cell washer is working properly, it should be tested at least once per week, by placing, in all positions, a tube containing a drop of IgG sensitised control cells plus one drop of AB serum. The tubes are then washed, AHG added, and the results read as per a normal test. All tubes should give equal strength positive reactions. If not, the cell washer should be taken out of service, cleaned, fresh saline placed in the reservoir and the quality control tests repeated. Only if satisfactory results are found in all tube positions can the washer be used. Records of these quality control tests must be kept (see also 'Guidelines for compatibility procedures in blood transfusion laboratories', see Sources of Additional Information for reference details).

APPLICATIONS OF THE INDIRECT ANTIGLOBULIN TEST (IAT)

Correctly performed, the IAT test is an extremely sensitive technique and is used extensively in blood group serology related to the following situations:

Red cell grouping

A patient's (or donor's) red cell sample is tested against a specific (IgG) antiserum (e.g. such as anti-Fy^a) to detect the presence of a particular antigen on the test red cell sample.

Controls: Positive and negative control red cell samples should be used for the grouping serum, i.e. which for anti-Fy^a would be an Fy(a+b+) sample for the positive control and an Fy(a-b+) sample for the negative control (see Section 5: Basic Serological Techniques and Controls). For AHG tube techniques, IgG sensitised red cells should be used to check all negative test results.

NOTE: The use of an AHG test for red cell grouping is less routinely used due to the increasing availability of monoclonal saline reactive sera.

Antibody screening (detection)

The patient's (or donor's) serum/plasma sample is tested against a small number (e.g. normally two) of phenotyped reagent red cell samples (specifically selected so that they express all of the major red cell antigens between them), to determine the presence of immune (irregular) alloantibodies.

Controls: Each of the antibody screening red cells used should be tested using a weak anti-Rh (usually an anti-D and/or anti-c) serum as a positive control and AB serum as a negative control. Additionally another weak antibody specificity such as an anti-Fy^a can be used to assure not only technique sensitivity but also to demonstrate integrity of antigen expression of the stored reagent red cells (an anti-Fy^a is frequently used for this purpose as Duffy antigens may deteriorate with storage). For AHG tube techniques, IgG sensitised red cells should be used to check all negative test results.

Antibody identification

If an antibody screening test is positive, then the serum/plasma should be tested by the IAT technique against a panel of specially selected phenotyped red cells to determine the specificity(ies) of the antibody(ies) present. Specific controls are not normally used, however the use of weak examples of antibodies testing in parallel, as mentioned above for antibody screening, can be used if required (e.g. a weak anti-D, anti-c, and/or anti-Fy^a). For AHG tube techniques, IgG sensitised red cells should be added to check all negative reactions.

Compatibility testing ('Crossmatching')

Donor red cells are tested against the patient's serum/plasma, to determine whether the donor red cells are compatible with the potential recipient, i.e. that the patient does not have an immune antibody active against an antigen present on the donor red cells. If the test is negative, the unit of red cells can be labelled and issued for transfusion to that patient (see Section 8: Pre-Transfusion Testing).

Controls: At least once per shift (or batch of tests, etc.) a positive control of a weak anti-D plus O R_1r cells and a negative control of AB serum plus O R_1r red cells, should be performed. This is used to control the reactivity of the AHG reagent. For AHG tube techniques, IgG sensitised red cells should be used to check all negative test results.

CAUSES OF FALSE POSITIVE RESULTS IN THE INDIRECT <u>TUBE</u> AHG TEST

a. Presence of particulate matter, dust, plastic particles, etc., in the tube.
b. Presence of substances in the saline that leads to non-specific agglutination of the red cells (e.g. colloidal silica or metal ions).
c. Poorly absorbed polyclonal AHG reagent, which will react with un-coated human red cells.
d. Cross-contamination from one tube to another, or from poorly cleaned cell washers.
e. Red cells with a positive direct antiglobulin test.
f. Over-centrifugation.
g. Failure to detect agglutination before washing the cells.
h. Wrong / incorrect LISS concentration (i.e. too low).

CAUSES OF FALSE NEGATIVE RESULTS IN THE INDIRECT <u>TUBE</u> AHG TEST

a. Inadequate washing of the red cells, i.e. as little as a 1 in 4,000 dilution of serum/plasma in saline is capable of neutralising an equivalent volume of AHG reagent.
b. Failure to add AHG reagent.
c. Inactive AHG reagent due to inadequate storage conditions, contamination with bacteria or serum, use after the reagent's expiry date, etc.
d. Loss of antigens from the red cell surface due to prolonged or inadequate sample/red cell storage.
e. Inactive serum/plasma due to inadequate storage conditions, e.g. repeated freezing and thawing, etc.
f. Inadequate incubation time or temperature.
g. Presence of fibrin clots; these will exude serum even after washing and will neutralise the AHG reagent.
h. Cross-contamination with other tubes (e.g. as when the tube is inverted against the finger, which is contaminated with serum or blood).
i. Un-buffered saline at too low a pH (antibodies elute from red cells at a low pH).
j. Excess antigen, i.e. too many red cells in the reaction mixture.
k. Leaving the cells too long before adding the AHG reagent (weakly bound antibodies may elute from the red cells) or after adding the AHG reagent (positive IATs, due to IgG coating, becoming weaker on standing).
l. Wrong / incorrect LISS concentration (i.e. too high).

Diagrammatic representation of the principle of the AHG test (not to scale)

INCUBATION
Mix and incubate the red cell and serum/plasma mixture.

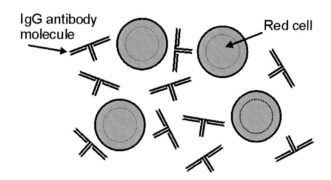

Antigen-antibody reaction (i.e. primary stage of agglutination). Some free antibody is also present.

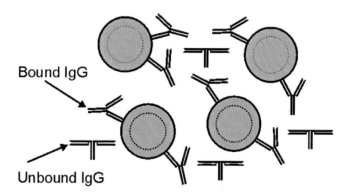

WASH RED CELLS TO REMOVE FREE (UNBOUND) IMMUNOGLOBULIN
After washing, the red cell bound antibody is still present, whereas excess (unbound) antibody has been removed.

ANTI-HUMAN GLOBULIN (AHG) REAGENT ADDED
Anti-human globulin molecules bind to the Fc portion of red cell bound antibody to form 'bridges', resulting in red cell agglutination.

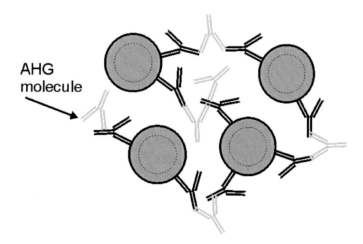

QUESTIONS - SECTION 6

1. Indicate and explain the main steps in an indirect (tube) antiglobulin test.

2. List five reasons why a false positive result may be obtained in an IAT.

3. List five reasons why a false negative result may be obtained in an IAT.

4. How do IgG sensitised red cells work in controlling the AHG test?

5. What is the difference between an IAT and a DAT?

6. What is the advantage of using a 'broad spectrum' AHG reagent?

7. What is the primary difference in the use of serum or plasma samples for the AHG test?

8. If no red cells are detected on the surface, within or at the bottom of a gel AHG test used for a crossmatch, what does this signify and why?

9. What should be added to each tube position of a cell washer to control its action?

10. What concentration of serum is capable of inhibiting AHG reagent added to a AHG test, resulting in a false negative result?

SECTION 7

ANTIBODY DETECTION AND IDENTIFICATION

WHY ARE BLOOD GROUP ANTIBODIES IMPORTANT?

Blood group antibodies of the ABO system are universally common, but those of the other blood group systems are only produced when red cells are transferred to a patient via a blood transfusion or a fetal red cell bleed during pregnancy. Theoretically, any of the antigens present on the transferred red cells which are not also present on the patient's own red cells may be recognised as foreign by the recipient's immune system and (atypical) antibody production stimulated. However, this does not routinely occur and antibody stimulation to any individual red cell antigen is dependant upon a number of factors including the immunogenicity of the individual antigen concerned, the amount and frequency of the stimulation involved and the factors related to the recipient's own immune response capability.

The 'clinical significance' of such antibodies varies with (for example) the blood group specificity / reactivity, reaction temperature, complement activating capability and amount (titre). Clinically significant antibodies are regarded as ones that react *in vitro* at 37°C by the AHG technique and are capable of causing either a transfusion reaction and/or HDFN (see Section 8: Pre-Transfusion Testing). Blood group antibodies are only important to the patient when they require a transfusion or are pregnant.

Alloantibodies and transfusion

When an individual is first stimulated to produce an antibody it takes some time for the immune system to be activated and possibly up to 3 months before the antibody becomes detectable. This is a primary response. However, if there is a second challenge by the same antigen then antibodies are produced rapidly, as the immune system has been primed; this is a secondary response. Initially in an immune response IgM antibodies are produced but class switching then occurs and IgG antibodies are produced in large numbers.

Transfusion provides an opportunity for antibody stimulation though the red cells that cause the antibody stimulation usually survive in the circulation normally, due to the delay in producing the immune response. If however a patient, already stimulated to produce a blood group antibody, is transfused with red cells carrying the corresponding antigen, these red cells may be destroyed by the pre-existing antibody. The effects of this transfusion reaction may vary from the 'barely detectable', through a range of conditions increasingly unpleasant for the patient, to possibly even death (see Section 9: Transfusion Reactions).

Serious transfusion reactions may result in the donor red cells being destroyed in the patient's circulation (intravascular) and/or sequestered via their reaction with macrophages in the liver and/or spleen (extravascular). It is therefore necessary to detect and identify any blood group antibodies in the potential recipient prior to transfusion, so that specifically selected antigen negative blood can be transfused and therefore avoid any possible red cell destruction and transfusion reaction.

An antibody screening (detection) test may be positive although the crossmatch would indicate that the cells being tested are compatible. This situation may occur due to the fact that the red cells used for antibody screening may be able to detect the presence of an antibody in the patient's serum/plasma better than using the donor's red cells. The red cells used for antibody screening are specially selected to have a homozygous expression ('double dose') for the important clinically significant antigens to

70

give maximal antigen expression. A weak antibody may fail to react with the donor cells if they only express a 'single dose' antigen, i.e. are heterozygous, but may react with the stronger antigen expressed on the screening cells ('antigen dosage' effects). In this situation, a negative cross-match does not necessarily indicate that the blood will be compatible if transfused and blood should not be transfused until a full antibody investigation has been performed. This should include 'antibody identification' tests, i.e. identification of the specificity of the blood group antibody, and if appropriate, selecting grouped donor red cells shown to lack the antigen corresponding to the antibody specificity (see Section 8: Pre-Transfusion Testing).

Alloantibodies and pregnancy

During pregnancy, and especially at delivery, fetal red cells can leak into the maternal circulation. If these red cells carry an antigen (or antigens) inherited from the father that are not found on the maternal red cells, these 'foreign' antigens may stimulate the mother to produce antibodies. Antibodies are not usually found in a first pregnancy, unless they are the result of a previous transfusion, as the usual time of stimulation is at delivery or in the third trimester of the pregnancy. The most common antibody produced in this way is anti-D, in D negative women. Other Rh antibodies, such as anti-c, and anti-K can also be stimulated this way.

Once stimulated, the IgG antibody crosses the placenta and is capable of destroying fetal red cells that carry the appropriate antigen, especially in subsequent pregnancies. It is therefore necessary to detect and determine the specificity of any such antibodies in the serum/plasma of pregnant women, i.e. to assess if the fetus will be at risk and/or for the provision of antigen negative blood should the mother and/or the baby require a transfusion. Further information can be obtained from 'Guidelines for blood grouping and red cell antibody testing during pregnancy', see Sources of Additional Information for reference details (see Section 11: Haemolytic Disease of the Fetus/Newborn).

ANTIBODY SCREENING (DETECTION)

The serum/plasma from a patient is tested against specifically selected red cell samples, called antibody screening red cells. Between 1%-3% of all hospital patients have atypical antibodies in their serum, stimulated either by a previous transfusion or pregnancy. The chance of being stimulated to produce an alloantibody increases with the number of transfusion and/or pregnancy events. The commonest antibody specificities encountered are anti-D (-C+D), -E, -K, -c, -Fy^a and -Jk^a.

The red cell samples used for antibody screening tests (usually either two or three) are specifically chosen to give good expression of all antigen specificities reactive with antibodies which are known to cause transfusion problems, i.e. antibodies which are clinically significant. The correct selection of these red cells is therefore essential and will involve the preferable use of red cells having homozygous expression for certain antigens; especially those known to show marked dosage effects, e.g. Kidd antigens (see Section 10: Other Blood Group Systems).

The 'Guidelines for pre-transfusion compatibility procedures in blood transfusion laboratories' identifies that, as a minimum, reagent red cells for antibody screening should express the following antigens:

C, c, D, E, e, K, k, Fy^a, Fy^b, Jk^a, Jk^b, S, s, M, N and Le^a

Reagent red cells, used for antibody screening, obtained from different donors should not be pooled in an attempt to achieve the required representation of antigens. In addition, it is recommended that apparent homozygous expression of the following antigens is desirable Jk^a, Jk^b, S, s, Fy^a, and Fy^b

Some commonly found antibodies are 'naturally acquired' (i.e. have not been stimulated as the result of a transfusion and/or pregnancy), do not react at $37^{\circ}C$ and are therefore not clinically significant (e.g. examples of anti-P_1, anti-Le^b, anti-I). Some antibodies may be significant if reactive at $37^{\circ}C$, but are often only reactive at lower temperatures (e.g. anti-M).

Antibody screening of blood donations

Antibody screening is carried out by an automated technique on the plasma samples taken with every blood donation to detect the presence of strong immune blood group antibodies. The purpose of this is to prevent a "minor" transfusion incompatibility, i.e. transfused antibody in the donor plasma destroying the (antigen positive) recipient's red cells. Donor blood found to contain antibodies reacting at temperatures below $37^{\circ}C$ or by enzyme techniques only is considered safe for transfusion, since the clinical effects of the transfusion of such antibodies will be negligible.

Additional, more sensitive antibody screening tests are performed on donations intended for fetal/neonatal transfusion, due to the small blood volume of these recipients to ensure that these donations are free of all clinically significant antibodies, including high titre anti-A and anti-B (see Section 13: Blood Donation Testing).

ANTIBODY IDENTIFICATION

Antibody identification is performed when an antibody detection test has been found to be positive. Essentially blood group antibody screening and identification are similar procedures since the same basic techniques are used, although a saline $20^{\circ}C$ technique and enzyme $37^{\circ}C$ technique may also be employed for antibody identification (especially where two or more antibody specificities are thought to be present).

Antibody identification techniques involve testing the patient's serum/plasma against known phenotyped red cell samples, though the difference is that instead of the 2-3 red cell samples used for antibody screening, a larger number of red cell samples are usually used for (initial) antibody identification, i.e. 9-11. This is called a red cell "panel". As a minimum the antibody identification panel should include the following antigen specificities:

C, C^w, c, D, E, e, K, k, Kp^a, Fy^a, Fy^b, Jk^a, Jk^b, S, s, Le^a, Le^b, M, N, P_1 and Lu^a

The panel cells used should meet guideline recommendations in being able to easily differentiate clinically significant antibodies which are most frequently encountered, e.g. anti-D, anti-c, anti-K, etc., by a distinct pattern of reactivity. Commonly encountered combinations of antibodies should also be differentiated, e.g. anti-D+K, anti-Le^a + Le^b, etc.

Knowledge of the typical reactivity of different antibody specificities (i.e. by which techniques and at what temperature they normally react), helps in the identification process; for example anti-P_1 works normally by saline techniques at $20^{\circ}C$; anti-Fy^a works by IAT but not by enzyme techniques at $37^{\circ}C$, etc.

Summary of expected antibody reactivity

ANTIBODY SPECIFICITIES	NORMAL REACTIVITY EXPECTED *
Anti-K, -k, -Jk^a, -Jk^b	Normally reactive at 37°C (by AHG and enzyme techniques) and not at 20°C
Anti-D, -C, -c, -E, -e	Normally reactive by AHG and enzyme techniques at 37°C (and not at 20°C), though some react as 'enzyme only'
Anti-Fy^a, -Fy^b, -S	Reactive at 37°C by AHG techniques only (not reactive by enzyme techniques)
Anti-P$_1$, -H, -I, -Lu^a, -Lu^b, -N, some anti-M	Normally reactive by saline techniques at temperatures up to 20°C (rarely at 37°C)
Anti-Le^a, -Le^b, some anti-M and anti-s	Possibly reactive at both 37°C and 20°C

* The use of the terms 'normally' and 'possibly' in the above table illustrate that variable reactivity has been described. See Section 10 for separate information regarding individual antibody specificities.

Interpretation of the results must be performed with care; it is not sufficient just to try to match the positive and negative results obtained with the positive and negative symbols shown on the panel's antigen profile. Clear-cut reactions with, where possible, at least two positive and two negative red cell samples are required to validate the specificity of every 'regularly' encountered blood group antibody specificity. This may not be possible for 'high frequency' (e.g. k, H, Kp^b, etc.) and 'low frequency' (e.g. Lu^a, Kp^a, etc.) antigens. Some antibody identification panels also contain a cord red cell sample, to enable the identification of anti-I and anti-HI specificities, since cord red cells are I negative, as well as being always Le(a-b-).

Some reactions may be due to the presence of more than one antibody specificity, whereas other results may represent specificities reacting only with homozygous (rather than heterozygous) red cell antigenic expression. It is essential to ensure when identifying an antibody specificity that the positive reactions obtained with the panel cells do not 'mask' the presence of another alloantibody specificity.

Antibody identification is relatively straightforward for patient's serum/plasma sample that contains a single antibody specificity. Some patients however, especially those who have been multiply transfused, may form two (or even more) antibody specificities. The serum/plasma from such patients may react with every red cell sample on the panel, but may give different patterns of reactivity in the different techniques and reaction temperatures used. By careful elimination of different specificities and the possible use of further selected panel cells, resolution of the components of complex antibody mixtures is usually possible. However, these tests would normally be performed only in recognised reference laboratories.

When the specificity of an antibody has been determined, it is normal to seek confirmation of the specificity by grouping the patient's red cells for the corresponding antigen, i.e. the person should be X negative for them to be able to produce anti-X.

List of antibodies most commonly found in patients

ANTIBODY SPECIFICITY	APPROXIMATE PERCENTAGE OF PATIENT'S SAMPLES POSITIVE
ANTI-D	0.3%
ANTI-C+D	0.2%
ANTI-D+E	0.06%
ANTI-E	0.5%
ANTI-c	0.1%
ANTI-K	0.4%
ANTI-Fy^a	0.04%
ANTI-Jk^a	0.02%
ANTI-S	0.01%

AUTOANTIBODIES AND IMMUNE HAEMOLYTIC ANAEMIAS

Red cell antibodies produced as a result of transfusion and/or pregnancy can cause either the destruction of red cells if incompatible blood is transfused, i.e. a haemolytic transfusion reaction (HTR), or the destruction of fetal red cells, i.e. Haemolytic Disease of the Fetus/Newborn (HDFN). Some patients may however produce autoantibodies, directed against their own red cells, which can lead to anaemia, i.e. Autoimmune Haemolytic Anaemia (AIHA). This is a relatively rare event but AIHA is frequently found in a patient secondary to other clinical disorders and may result from a variety of possible causes. In addition, some patients may produce antibodies that react with their own red cells if they are taking certain drugs, which results in drug-associated, or 'drug-induced' haemolytic anaemia. This can occur due to a variety of processes that result in the patient's red cells being recognised as 'foreign' by the patient's immune system, associated with the presence of a drug. The AIHAs are recognised by the combination of having the usual signs of anaemia (low haemoglobin) together with a positive direct antiglobulin test (DAT), resulting from the *in vivo* reaction of autoantibody and patient's red cells. Both auto-immune and drug associated immune destruction of platelets can also occur

Additional specialist serological tests can be performed on blood samples from these patients. This is especially true when the autoantibody reacts with all cells samples as well as the patient's own, since these positive reactions may be masking the presence of one or more alloantibodies, which must be identified prior to any transfusion. As a result, the investigation and crossmatching of blood for AIHA cases is normally performed by reference laboratories. Transfusions should be avoided if other treatments can be used. If a transfusion is required and the antibody screen is negative, blood should be selected and cross-matched in the normal manner. If however, the antibody detection tests are positive, then the additional tests referred to above need to be employed to exclude the presence of alloantibodies which may also be present with and masked by unbound autoantibody free in the patient's serum/plasma. These specialist techniques involve alloadsorption and possibly elution, and are normally performed by reference laboratories (see also 'Guidelines for the pre-transfusion compatibility procedures in blood transfusion laboratories', see Sources of Additional Information for reference details).

The practice of selecting blood for patients with a positive DAT and a positive antibody screen as "the least incompatible" units by virtue of reaction strength in the crossmatch is <u>not</u> an acceptable procedure. Autoantibodies in the patient's serum/plasma can mask the presence of alloantibodies and it is these that cause rapid destruction of transfused red cells, which might exacerbate rather than help the patient's condition (see Section 12: Immune Haemolytic Anaemias).

QUESTIONS - SECTION 7

1. Explain the difference between an 'alloantibody' and an 'autoantibody'.

2. List the most commonly identified IgG antibody specificities to be found in patient's serum/plasma.

3. Why is homozygosity of antigenic expression, for certain antigens, important for antibody screening cells?

4. List the antigens that should be present on red cells used for antibody detection.

5. Which antibody specificities are produced principally via pregnancy?

6. Why is the antibody detection test potentially more important than the crossmatch for detecting alloantibodies?

7. What percentage of patients is likely to have a pre-formed alloantibody?

8. What does a positive crossmatch together with a negative antibody detection test result signify?

9. Outline the process by which antibodies are stimulated by pregnancy.

10. Which blood donations are given additional (more sensitive) antibody screening tests?

ASSIGNMENT

Using data collected from your Blood Bank records, calculate the frequency of a 'positive antibody screening test'. If possible, divide these into pre-transfusion and antenatal patients and identify the frequency in the two groups. Is there a significant difference between them, and if so, can you suggest why?

From your Blood Bank records, list the antibody specificities identified from these positive antibody screen tests. Is there a significant difference between the specificities found in the two groups of patients, and if so, can you suggest why?

ANTIBODY IDENTIFICATION EXERCISE

The 'Guidelines for compatibility procedures in blood transfusion laboratories' (2004) makes the following statements regarding antibody identification:

1. The specificity of the antibody should only be assigned when it is reactive with at least two examples of reagent red cells carrying the antigen and non-reactive with at least two examples of reagent red cells lacking the antigen. Note that, wherever possible, the presence of anti-Jk^a, anti-Jk^b, anti-S, anti-s, anti-Fy^a and anti-Fy^b should be excluded using red cells having homozygous expression of the relevant antigen (section 7.7.2 of the Guideline).

2. When one antibody specificity has been identified, it is essential that the presence of additional clinically significant antibodies is not missed. Multiple antibodies can only be confirmed by choosing cells that are antigen negative for the recognised specificity but positive for other antigens to which clinically significant antibodies may arise (section 7.7.4 of the Guideline).

RESULTS

You are provided with a series of antibody identification results, using IAT and enzyme (papain) techniques at 37°C from 12 patients.

Notes:
Techniques: Whilst the use of IAT and enzyme techniques might not reflect a normal practical situation within your laboratory, it is used here with the specific intention of providing information to help you to work out the antibody specificity concerned.
Antibody identification panel: The panel sheet has been put together specifically for the purpose of this exercise and is not intended to reflect an actual antibody identification panel for use in a laboratory situation, neither should it be taken as suggesting an ideal format.
All antibody identification cells are group O.
All 12 patients have a negative DAT and their 'auto' (normally recorded on a separate row at the bottom of the panel sheet) has therefore been omitted to save space.

QUESTIONS

You are required in this exercise to:

1. Identify the probable antibody specificity (or specificities) present in each of the 12 samples using the panel results provided.

2. Provide information as to the presence of any 'masked' antibody specificities.
   Identify any antibody specificities against low frequency antigens (e.g. anti-Lu^a, -Kp^a, -C^w, etc.) that cannot be excluded and describe how you would deal with this situation.
   Identify any instance where section 7.7.2 of the Guidelines (see above) has <u>not</u> been met (i.e. two homozygous cells are non-reactive for each of the excluded specificities). Identify what you would do serologically to resolve the problem.

3. Provide information as to the type of blood that you would provide for the patient.

Note

This exercise is designed to provide specific examples relating to the principles of antibody identification. It is <u>strongly</u> recommended that you should receive further instruction on this subject from colleagues and additional experience / practice with regard to the interpretation of antibody identification panels.

Patient 1

	Rh	D	C	E	c	e	M	N	S	s	P₁	Lu a	Lu b	K	k	Kp a	Kp b	Le a	Le b	Fy a	Fy b	Jk a	Jk b	IAT	Enz
1	$R_1^wR_1$	+	+	-	-	+	+	+	+	-	-	-	+	-	+	-	+	+	-	+	-	-	+	3	3
2	R_1R_1	+	+	-	-	+	+	-	-	+	4	-	+	+	+	-	+	-	+	-	+	+	-	3	3
3	R_2R_2	+	-	+	+	-	-	+	-	+	-	-	+	-	+	-	+	-	+	+	+	+	-	3	3
4	r'r	-	+	-	+	+	-	+	+	-	2	-	+	-	+	-	+	-	+	-	+	-	+	3	3
5	r''r	-	-	+	+	+	+	-	+	-	-	-	+	-	+	-	+	-	+	-	+	+	-	0	0
6	rr	-	-	-	+	+	+	+	+	+	2	-	+	+	+	-	+	-	+	-	+	+	+	0	0
7	rr	-	-	-	+	+	-	+	+	-	1	-	+	-	+	+	+	-	-	+	-	-	+	0	0
8	rr	-	-	-	+	+	+	-	+	+	3	+	+	+	+	-	+	+	-	+	+	+	-	0	0
9	rr	-	-	-	+	+	-	+	-	+	-	-	+	-	+	-	+	-	+	+	-	-	+	0	0
10	rr	-	-	-	+	+	+	+	-	+	3	-	+	+	+	-	+	-	+	+	-	-	+	0	0

Patient 2

	Rh	D	C	E	c	e	M	N	S	s	P₁	Lu a	Lu b	K	k	Kp a	Kp b	Le a	Le b	Fy a	Fy b	Jk a	Jk b	IAT	Enz
1	$R_1^wR_1$	+	+	-	-	+	+	+	+	-	-	-	+	-	+	-	+	+	-	+	-	-	+	0	0
2	R_1R_1	+	+	-	-	+	+	-	-	+	4	-	+	+	+	-	+	-	+	-	+	+	-	4	4
3	R_2R_2	+	-	+	+	-	-	+	-	+	-	-	+	-	+	-	+	-	+	+	+	+	-	0	0
4	r'r	-	+	-	+	+	-	+	+	-	2	-	+	-	+	-	+	-	+	-	+	-	+	0	0
5	r''r	-	-	+	+	+	+	-	+	-	-	-	+	-	+	-	+	-	+	-	+	+	-	0	0
6	rr	-	-	-	+	+	+	+	+	+	2	-	+	+	+	-	+	-	-	+	-	+	+	4	4
7	rr	-	-	-	+	+	-	+	+	-	1	-	+	-	+	-	+	+	-	-	+	-	+	0	0
8	rr	-	-	-	+	+	+	-	+	+	3	+	+	+	+	-	+	+	-	+	+	+	-	4	4
9	rr	-	-	-	+	+	-	+	-	+	-	-	+	-	+	-	+	-	+	+	-	-	+	0	0
10	rr	-	-	-	+	+	+	+	-	+	3	-	+	+	+	-	+	-	+	+	-	-	+	4	4

Patient 3

	Rh	D	C	E	c	e	M	N	S	s	P₁	Lu a	Lu b	K	k	Kp a	Kp b	Le a	Le b	Fy a	Fy b	Jk a	Jk b	IAT	Enz
1	$R_1^wR_1$	+	+	-	-	+	+	+	+	-	-	-	+	-	+	-	+	+	-	+	-	-	+	0	0
2	R_1R_1	+	+	-	-	+	+	-	-	+	4	-	+	+	+	-	+	-	+	-	+	+	-	0	0
3	R_2R_2	+	-	+	+	-	-	+	-	+	-	-	+	-	+	-	+	-	+	+	+	+	-	2	4
4	r'r	-	+	-	+	+	-	+	+	-	2	-	+	-	+	-	+	-	+	-	+	-	+	2	4
5	r''r	-	-	+	+	+	+	-	+	-	-	-	+	-	+	-	+	-	+	-	+	+	-	2	4
6	rr	-	-	-	+	+	+	+	+	+	2	-	+	+	+	-	+	-	+	-	+	+	+	2	4
7	rr	-	-	-	+	+	-	+	+	-	1	-	+	-	+	+	+	-	-	+	-	-	+	2	4
8	rr	-	-	-	+	+	+	-	+	+	3	+	+	+	+	-	+	+	-	+	+	+	-	2	4
9	rr	-	-	-	+	+	-	+	-	+	-	-	+	-	+	-	+	-	+	+	-	-	+	2	4
10	rr	-	-	-	+	+	+	+	-	+	3	-	+	+	+	-	+	-	+	+	-	-	+	2	4

Patient 4

	Rh	D	C	E	c	e	M	N	S	s	P₁	Lu a	Lu b	K	k	Kp a	Kp b	Le a	Le b	Fy a	Fy b	Jk a	Jk b	IAT	Enz
1	$R_1^wR_1$	+	+	-	-	+	+	+	+	-	-	-	+	-	+	-	+	+	-	+	-	-	+	3	0
2	R_1R_1	+	+	-	-	+	+	-	-	+	4	-	+	+	+	-	+	-	+	-	+	+	-	0	0
3	R_2R_2	+	-	+	+	-	-	+	-	+	-	-	+	-	+	-	+	-	+	+	+	+	-	3	0
4	r'r	-	+	-	+	+	-	+	+	-	2	-	+	-	+	-	+	-	+	-	+	-	+	0	0
5	r''r	-	-	+	+	+	+	-	+	-	-	-	+	-	+	-	+	-	+	-	+	+	-	0	0
6	rr	-	-	-	+	+	+	+	+	+	2	-	+	+	+	-	+	-	-	+	-	+	+	3	0
7	rr	-	-	-	+	+	-	+	+	-	1	-	+	-	+	-	+	+	-	-	+	-	+	0	0
8	rr	-	-	-	+	+	+	-	+	+	3	+	+	+	+	-	+	+	-	+	+	+	-	3	0
9	rr	-	-	-	+	+	-	+	-	+	-	-	+	-	+	-	+	-	+	+	-	-	+	3	0
10	rr	-	-	-	+	+	+	+	-	+	3	-	+	+	+	-	+	-	+	+	-	-	+	3	0

Patient 5

	Rh	D	C	E	c	e	M	N	S	s	P₁	Lu a	Lu b	K	k	Kp a	Kp b	Le a	Le b	Fy a	Fy b	Jk a	Jk b	IAT	Enz
1	R₁wR₁	+	+	-	-	+	+	+	+	-	-	-	+	-	+	-	+	+	-	+	-	-	+	2	0
2	R₁R₁	+	+	-	-	+	+	-	-	+	4	-	+	+	+	-	+	-	+	-	+	+	-	4	0
3	R₂R₂	+	-	+	+	-	-	+	-	+	-	-	+	-	+	-	+	-	+	+	+	+	-	0	0
4	r'r	-	+	-	+	+	-	+	+	-	2	-	+	-	+	-	+	-	+	-	+	-	+	0	0
5	r"r	-	-	+	+	+	+	-	+	-	-	-	+	-	+	-	+	-	+	-	+	+	-	4	0
6	rr	-	-	-	+	+	+	+	+	+	2	-	+	+	+	-	+	-	-	+	-	+	+	2	0
7	rr	-	-	-	+	+	-	+	+	-	1	-	+	-	+	-	+	+	-	-	+	-	+	0	0
8	rr	-	-	-	+	+	+	-	+	+	3	+	+	+	+	-	+	+	-	+	+	+	-	4	0
9	rr	-	-	-	+	+	-	+	-	+	-	-	+	-	+	-	+	-	+	+	-	-	+	0	0
10	rr	-	-	-	+	+	+	+	-	+	3	-	+	+	+	-	+	-	+	+	-	-	+	4	0

Patient 6

	Rh	D	C	E	c	e	M	N	S	s	P₁	Lu a	Lu b	K	k	Kp a	Kp b	Le a	Le b	Fy a	Fy b	Jk a	Jk b	IAT	Enz
1	R₁wR₁	+	+	-	-	+	+	+	+	-	-	-	+	-	+	-	+	+	-	+	-	-	+	2	3
2	R₁R₁	+	+	-	-	+	+	-	-	+	4	-	+	+	+	-	+	-	+	-	+	+	-	0	0
3	R₂R₂	+	-	+	+	-	-	+	-	+	-	-	+	-	+	-	+	-	+	+	+	+	-	0	0
4	r'r	-	+	-	+	+	-	+	+	-	2	-	+	-	+	-	+	-	+	-	+	-	+	2	2
5	r"r	-	-	+	+	+	+	-	+	-	-	-	+	-	+	-	+	-	+	-	+	+	-	0	0
6	rr	-	-	-	+	+	+	+	+	+	2	-	+	+	+	-	+	-	-	+	-	+	+	1	2
7	rr	-	-	-	+	+	-	+	+	-	1	-	+	-	+	-	+	+	-	-	+	-	+	2	3
8	rr	-	-	-	+	+	+	-	+	+	3	+	+	+	+	-	+	+	-	+	+	+	-	0	0
9	rr	-	-	-	+	+	-	+	-	+	-	-	+	-	+	-	+	-	+	+	-	-	+	2	3
10	rr	-	-	-	+	+	+	+	-	+	3	-	+	+	+	-	+	-	+	+	-	-	+	2	3

Patient 7

	Rh	D	C	E	c	e	M	N	S	s	P₁	Lu a	Lu b	K	k	Kp a	Kp b	Le a	Le b	Fy a	Fy b	Jk a	Jk b	IAT	Enz
1	R₁wR₁	+	+	-	-	+	+	+	+	-	-	-	+	-	+	-	+	+	-	+	-	-	+	0	0
2	R₁R₁	+	+	-	-	+	+	-	-	+	4	-	+	+	+	-	+	-	+	-	+	+	-	3	3
3	R₂R₂	+	-	+	+	-	-	+	-	+	-	-	+	-	+	-	+	-	+	+	+	+	-	1	2
4	r'r	-	+	-	+	+	-	+	+	-	2	-	+	-	+	-	+	-	+	-	+	-	+	3	3
5	r"r	-	-	+	+	+	+	-	+	-	-	-	+	-	+	-	+	-	+	-	+	+	-	2	2
6	rr	-	-	-	+	+	+	+	+	+	2	-	+	+	+	-	+	-	-	+	-	+	+	0	0
7	rr	-	-	-	+	+	-	+	+	-	1	-	+	-	+	-	+	+	-	-	+	-	+	0	0
8	rr	-	-	-	+	+	+	-	+	+	3	+	+	+	+	-	+	+	-	+	+	+	-	0	0
9	rr	-	-	-	+	+	-	+	-	+	-	-	+	-	+	-	+	-	+	+	-	-	+	2	2
10	rr	-	-	-	+	+	+	+	-	+	3	-	+	+	+	-	+	-	+	+	-	-	+	1	3

Patient 8

	Rh	D	C	E	c	e	M	N	S	s	P₁	Lu a	Lu b	K	k	Kp a	Kp b	Le a	Le b	Fy a	Fy b	Jk a	Jk b	IAT	Enz
1	R₁wR₁	+	+	-	-	+	+	+	+	-	-	-	+	-	+	-	+	+	-	+	-	-	+	2	3
2	R₁R₁	+	+	-	-	+	+	-	-	+	4	-	+	+	+	-	+	-	+	-	+	+	-	2	3
3	R₂R₂	+	-	+	+	-	-	+	-	+	-	-	+	-	+	-	+	-	+	+	+	+	-	0	0
4	r'r	-	+	-	+	+	-	+	+	-	2	-	+	-	+	-	+	-	+	-	+	-	+	2	3
5	r"r	-	-	+	+	+	+	-	+	-	-	-	+	-	+	-	+	-	+	-	+	+	-	2	3
6	rr	-	-	-	+	+	+	+	+	+	2	-	+	+	+	-	+	-	-	+	-	+	+	2	3
7	rr	-	-	-	+	+	-	+	+	-	1	-	+	-	+	-	+	+	-	-	+	-	+	2	3
8	rr	-	-	-	+	+	+	-	+	+	3	+	+	+	+	-	+	+	-	+	+	+	-	2	3
9	rr	-	-	-	+	+	-	+	-	+	-	-	+	-	+	-	+	-	+	+	-	-	+	2	3
10	rr	-	-	-	+	+	+	+	-	+	3	-	+	+	+	-	+	-	+	+	-	-	+	2	3

Patient 9

	Rh	D	C	E	c	e	M	N	S	s	P1	Lu a	Lu b	K	k	Kp a	Kp b	Le a	Le b	Fy a	Fy b	Jk a	Jk b	IAT	Enz
1	R₁ʷR₁	+	+	-	-	+	+	+	+	-		-	+	-	+	-	+	+	-	+	-	-	+	3	0
2	R₁R₁	+	+	-	-	+	+	-	-	+	4	-	+	+	+	-	+	-	+	-	+	+	-	0	0
3	R₂R₂	+	-	+	+	-	-	+	-	+		-	+	-	+	-	+	-	+	+	+	+	-	0	0
4	r′r	-	+	-	+	+	-	+	+	-	2	-	+	-	+	-	+	-	+	-	+	-	+	2	0
5	r″r	-	-	+	+	+	+	-	+	-		-	+	-	+	-	+	-	+	-	+	+	-	3	0
6	rr	-	-	-	+	+	+	+	+	+	2	-	+	+	+	-	+	-	-	+	-	+	+	1	0
7	rr	-	-	-	+	+	-	+	+	-	1	-	+	-	+	-	+	+	-	+	-	+	-	3	0
8	rr	-	-	-	+	+	+	-	+	+	3	+	+	+	+	-	+	+	-	+	+	+	-	1	0
9	rr	-	-	-	+	+	-	+	-	+		-	+	-	+	-	+	-	+	+	-	-	+	0	0
10	rr	-	-	-	+	+	+	+	-	+	3	-	+	+	+	-	+	-	+	+	-	-	+	0	0

Patient 10

	Rh	D	C	E	c	e	M	N	S	s	P1	Lu a	Lu b	K	k	Kp a	Kp b	Le a	Le b	Fy a	Fy b	Jk a	Jk b	IAT	Enz
1	R₁ʷR₁	+	+	-	-	+	+	+	+	-		-	+	-	+	-	+	+	-	+	-	-	+	0	0
2	R₁R₁	+	+	-	-	+	+	-	-	+	4	-	+	+	+	-	+	-	+	-	+	+	-	2	2
3	R₂R₂	+	-	+	+	-	-	+	-	+		-	+	-	+	-	+	-	+	+	+	+	-	0	0
4	r′r	-	+	-	+	+	-	+	+	-	2	-	+	-	+	-	+	-	+	-	+	-	+	1	2
5	r″r	-	-	+	+	+	+	-	+	-		-	+	-	+	-	+	-	+	-	+	+	-	0	0
6	rr	-	-	-	+	+	+	+	+	+	2	-	+	+	+	-	+	-	-	+	-	+	+	1	2
7	rr	-	-	-	+	+	-	+	+	-	1	-	+	-	+	-	+	+	-	+	-	+	-	1	1
8	rr	-	-	-	+	+	+	-	+	+	3	+	+	+	+	-	+	+	-	+	+	+	-	2	2
9	rr	-	-	-	+	+	-	+	-	+		-	+	-	+	-	+	-	+	+	-	-	+	0	0
10	rr	-	-	-	+	+	+	+	-	+	3	-	+	+	+	-	+	-	+	+	-	-	+	2	2

Patient 11

	Rh	D	C	E	c	e	M	N	S	s	P1	Lu a	Lu b	K	k	Kp a	Kp b	Le a	Le b	Fy a	Fy b	Jk a	Jk b	IAT	Enz
1	R₁ʷR₁	+	+	-	-	+	+	+	+	-		-	+	-	+	-	+	+	-	+	-	-	+	3	4
2	R₁R₁	+	+	-	-	+	+	-	-	+	4	-	+	+	+	-	+	-	+	-	+	+	-	3	4
3	R₂R₂	+	-	+	+	-	-	+	-	+		-	+	-	+	-	+	-	+	+	+	+	-	3	4
4	r′r	-	+	-	+	+	-	+	+	-	2	-	+	-	+	-	+	-	+	-	+	-	+	0	0
5	r″r	-	-	+	+	+	+	-	+	-		-	+	-	+	-	+	-	+	-	+	+	-	0	0
6	rr	-	-	-	+	+	+	+	+	+	2	-	+	+	+	-	+	-	-	+	-	+	+	2	0
7	rr	-	-	-	+	+	-	+	+	-	1	-	+	-	+	-	+	+	-	+	-	+	-	0	0
8	rr	-	-	-	+	+	+	-	+	+	3	+	+	+	+	-	+	+	-	+	+	+	-	2	0
9	rr	-	-	-	+	+	-	+	-	+		-	+	-	+	-	+	-	+	+	-	-	+	2	0
10	rr	-	-	-	+	+	+	+	-	+	3	-	+	+	+	-	+	-	+	+	-	-	+	2	0

Patient 12

	Rh	D	C	E	c	e	M	N	S	s	P1	Lu a	Lu b	K	k	Kp a	Kp b	Le a	Le b	Fy a	Fy b	Jk a	Jk b	IAT	Enz
1	R₁ʷR₁	+	+	-	-	+	+	+	+	-		-	+	-	+	-	+	+	-	+	-	-	+	0	0
2	R₁R₁	+	+	-	-	+	+	-	-	+	4	-	+	+	+	-	+	-	+	-	+	+	-	2	2
3	R₂R₂	+	-	+	+	-	-	+	-	+		-	+	-	+	-	+	-	+	+	+	+	-	2	2
4	r′r	-	+	-	+	+	-	+	+	-	2	-	+	-	+	-	+	-	+	-	+	-	+	0	0
5	r″r	-	-	+	+	+	+	-	+	-		-	+	-	+	-	+	-	+	-	+	+	-	2	2
6	rr	-	-	-	+	+	+	+	+	+	2	-	+	+	+	-	+	-	-	+	-	+	+	0	0
7	rr	-	-	-	+	+	-	+	+	-	1	-	+	-	+	-	+	+	-	+	-	+	-	0	0
8	rr	-	-	-	+	+	+	-	+	+	3	+	+	+	+	-	+	+	-	+	+	+	-	2	2
9	rr	-	-	-	+	+	-	+	-	+		-	+	-	+	-	+	-	+	+	-	-	+	0	0
10	rr	-	-	-	+	+	+	+	-	+	3	-	+	+	+	-	+	-	+	+	-	-	+	0	0

SECTION 8

PRE-TRANSFUSION TESTING

NOTE: This section should be read in conjunction with the 'Guidelines for compatibility procedures in blood transfusion laboratories' (see 'Sources of Additional Information' for reference details).

The techniques described in the preceding sections can be used in the following routine blood bank tests, which are carried out to ensure that blood provided for transfusion is compatible with the patient.

The pre-transfusion laboratory procedure should consist of the following elements:
- Checking the records (manual and/or computer) for any previous grouping and/or antibody detection (screening) results.
- Performing ABO and D grouping of the patient's blood sample.
- Performing an antibody detection (screening) test on the patient's blood sample (or mother in the case of neonatal transfusion) which, in the event of a positive screen, should be followed by antibody identification.
- Selection of blood.
- Crossmatching the patient's serum/plasma against the donor's red cells, or using an electronic issue system.

The overall procedure should, if performed correctly, detect both of the following:
- ABO incompatibilities between donor and recipient.
- Atypical IgG antibodies in the patient's serum/plasma.

NOTE: It is essential to:
- Check the details provided on both the blood sample and request form to ensure that the correct sample is used.
- Write out the work sheet before setting up any tests.
- Record the results directly onto the work sheet.
- Have the results checked by another scientist.
- Record the batch numbers of all reagents used.
- Ensure that reagents are 'in date'.
- Sign and date the worksheet and file it safely, as it must be kept for 30 years

ABO GROUPING

Red cell group use: IgM monoclonal anti-A and anti-B (the use of anti-A,B is optional).
Reverse group use: A_1, B and frequently O cells (the use of A_2 cells is optional).

A negative control of the patient's serum/plasma reacted with either the patient's own red cells or group O red cells. If no reliable serum group can be obtained, the cell group should be repeated.

Controls:
React each grouping antisera used with each red cell sample used (i.e. in a 'checkerboard' manner). A reagent control may also be required as recommended by the reagent manufacturer.

Rh D GROUPING

Rh D grouping should be performed using two IgM monoclonal anti-D reagents that should not detect category DVI partial D types (see Section 4: The Rh Blood Group System). An IAT (a 'weak D' test) should <u>not</u> be used for Rh D typing.

Controls:
React each anti-D grouping antisera used with D positive (R_1r) and D negative (rr) red cells. A reagent control may also be required as recommended by the reagent manufacturer.

The ABO and D grouping results should be verified against previous results for the patient if available. Any grouping discrepancies should be resolved prior to transfusion.

ANTIBODY SCREENING (DETECTION)

To detect atypical red cell antibodies, the patient's serum/plasma should be tested by an IAT against two or three antibody screening cells (an enzyme test is not required). If a positive result is obtained, i.e. indicating the presence of a potentially clinically significant antibody, the specificity(ies) of the antibody(ies) must be identified, so that antigen negative blood can be selected for the patient if required (see Section 7: Antibody Detection and Identification).

CROSSMATCHING

The potential recipient's serum/plasma should be tested against a red cell sample obtained from each of the donations intended for transfusion to that patient. If no atypical antibodies are detected in the antibody screen and there is no history of antibodies having been present in the past, an "immediate spin" crossmatch technique may be used to ensure that there is no gross incompatibility (e.g. ABO) between the patient's serum/plasma and the donor's red cells.

An IAT cross-match technique should be performed, though electronic issue of blood may be used if specific criteria are fulfilled. If an antibody has been detected, an IAT crossmatch technique must be used. After incubation at 37°C the IAT test must be inspected for agglutination and/or haemolysis before washing the cells and adding the AHG reagent. If agglutination, haemolysis or a positive IAT result is found, the blood is incompatible and cannot be used for transfusion.

Crossmatching procedures within hospital blood banks are invariably linked to a 'maximum surgical blood order schedule' (MSBOS) system. This is a scheme, agreed with hospital medical staff, which lists the number of units of blood that should be routinely (pre-operatively) crossmatched for elective surgical procedures. The schedule is based on a retrospective analysis of actual blood use for different surgical procedures. It attempts to match the amount of blood ordered to the amount of blood actually used (see also 'Guidelines for implementation of a maximum surgical blood order schedule', see Sources of Additional Information for reference details).

Emergency crossmatching

In an emergency, when time does not allow all the above tests to be performed, the guidelines recommend that an antibody screen be performed, in addition to the ABO and D typing. If the antibody screen is negative it is not necessary to carry out an IAT crossmatch. The blood can be issued on the basis of the group and screening results. Only in rare instances should blood be issued without any tests being performed; there is usually time to perform at least an ABO and D group on the patient and issue ABO and Rh D compatible units. In such circumstances, the antibody screen and IAT crossmatch can be performed in retrospect.

A single saline rapid (tube) test to detect ABO incompatibility has been shown to have a limited sensitivity. The incubation period identified in local procedures for such 'immediate spin emergency crossmatches' should be validated and adhered to, otherwise the somewhat limited sensitivity of this technique is restricted even further.

Electronic (computer) issue of blood

Increasingly, 'computer issuing' is now being more widely used to provide blood for patients. This procedure involves the ABO and D grouping of the patient and the screening of their serum/plasma for the presence of immune $37^{\circ}C$ alloantibodies using automated techniques. If the grouping results are found to be the same as those obtained with a previous sample and there is a negative antibody detection test, blood of the same ABO and D group is issued by a computer programme, without a serological crossmatch having been performed. NOTE: This system cannot be used for patients whose serum/plasma is known, or has been known, to contain a clinically significant red cell alloantibody or the grouping results are equivocal.

This method of blood selection and issue requires the use of a validated automated system for confirmed ABO and D grouping and antibody screening, which includes positive sample identification and electronic data transfer of results. In addition, the computer software used for the system must be validated to ensure that the issue of ABO incompatible blood is prevented. The validity of the donor's ABO and D groups are assured by the supplying Blood Centre and as such does not require confirmation. See also 'Guidelines for compatibility procedures in blood transfusion laboratories' and the 'Guidelines for blood bank computing' (see Sources of Additional Information for reference details).

TYPE AND SCREEN

For many surgical procedures it is not necessary to have cross-matched blood immediately available for the patient. Therefore, in such cases, the patient's blood sample may be tested for ABO and D groups and antibody screened only, a "type and screen" procedure.

In such cases, should the patient subsequently need blood quickly, by knowing the patient's blood group and the fact that their antibody screen is negative, blood can be provided by an electronic issue or immediate-spin cross-match, in the confident knowledge that the blood will be compatible.

If the antibody screen is however found to be positive, then the antibody specificity must be identified and, if clinically significant, blood which is negative for the appropriate antigen(s) should be obtained (as appropriate) and crossmatched by IAT.

The pre-transfusion investigation of a patient's blood sample

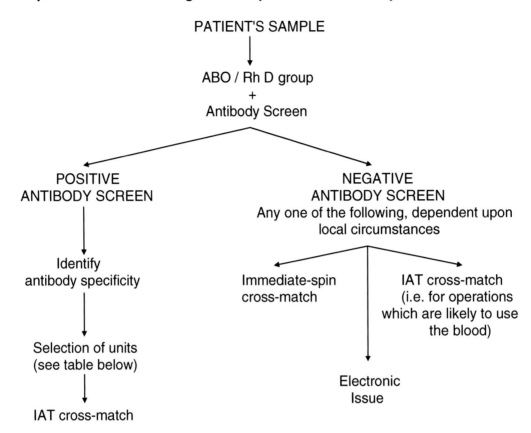

SELECTION OF BLOOD AND BLOOD COMPONENTS FOR TRANSFUSION

Each blood bank should have its own local policies for the selection and issue of blood and blood components, based on published guidelines. All staff must ensure that they are familiar with these policies. This is especially true for the use of certain specialised products (e.g. gamma-irradiated) and the transfusion of specific patient groups (e.g. infants and neonates) and the management of transfused patients with a clinically significant antibody. See the section Sources of Additional Information for reference details of the various guidelines on the use of fresh frozen plasma, platelets and red cells and specialised products, together with guidelines for the transfusion of specific patient groups and the management of transfused patients.

CLINICALLY SIGNIFICANT ANTIBODIES

Antibodies that give rise to the accelerated destruction of red cells following a transfusion, or cause HDFN, are considered clinically significant. Not all red cell antibodies cause *in vivo* cell destruction and there is sufficient evidence to show that alloantibodies that fail to react *in vitro* at 37°C, i.e. "cold reacting" alloantibodies, can be regarded as being not clinically significant.

The guidelines on pre-transfusion testing state that 'for patients with clinically significant antibodies blood should be selected which has been tested and found negative for the relevant antigen'. Blood for patients with a clinically significant alloantibody must not be selected on the basis of a negative IAT crossmatch result alone. If the antibodies are not clinically significant, it is not necessary to select antigen negative blood. Blood of the same ABO and D type as the patient should be selected for compatibility testing and 'IAT cross-match compatible blood' supplied for transfusion.

The following table (taken from the 'Guidelines for compatibility procedures in blood transfusion laboratories', see the section Sources of Additional Information for reference details), identifies what blood should be selected for patients with different antibody specificities.

Cold reacting antibodies and the selection of blood for transfusion

There is no evidence that cold reacting antibodies cause clinically significant *in vivo* destruction of red cells that carry the corresponding antigen, even when patients are subjected to hypothermia during surgery. If anti-P_1, -A_1, -Le^a, -Le^b, -Lu^a or -N reacting by an indirect antiglobulin technique is detected, it is unlikely that it will be reactive at strict 37°C. In this situation, if units of the same ABO and D type as the patient are selected, compatible units can normally be found without difficulty by using a 'pre-warmed' crossmatch technique. This involves warming the patient's serum/plasma and the donor red cells to 37°C prior to mixing them together and incubating at 37°C. This ensures that, if it happens, the reaction between antibody and antigen occurs strictly at 37°C and that there is no 'cooler incubation period' at the start of the incubation. At the end of the incubation period, the cells should be washed, or the microcolumn centrifuged immediately.

The use of anti-IgG in the AHG technique will further reduce the number of 'unwanted' cold reacting antibodies detected. Even if weakly reactive using pre-warmed techniques, it is rare that suitable compatible blood cannot be found for antibodies such as anti-P_1, -Le^a, -N and -Le^b. Crossmatching at 37°C will not affect the detection of ABO incompatibility (assuming sufficient incubation time is allowed).

Even those antibodies that react weakly in pre-warmed *in vitro* tests, rarely cause problems in finding suitable blood. For example, the P_1 antigen expression on red cells varies, and potent examples of anti-P_1 will often only react at 37°C with cells with a strong P_1 antigen. In addition, many examples of anti-Le^b that react by IAT with group O screening or panel cells, will fail to react with group A, B or AB cells as they are in fact anti-Le^{bH}, requiring both Le and H to be present on the red cells. Therefore if units of the patient's own ABO blood group are selected no incompatibility will be found on crossmatching.

Other antibody specificities of limited clinical significance in transfusion

Anti-C^w and anti-Kp^a are sometimes found in the absence of other alloantibodies. As these antibodies are of doubtful clinical significance and the incidence of the corresponding antigens is low (about 2% for both antigens), there is no need to select C^w negative or Kp^a negative blood. For anti-C^w, selecting Rh C negative blood is sufficient but for Kp^a it is only necessary to select blood of the same ABO and D type as the patient for crossmatching by IAT.

If there is any doubt about the reactivity of an antibody or its clinical significance, samples can be referred to a reference laboratory for testing, as well as for obtaining advice about the selection and testing of appropriate units for crossmatching and transfusion.

Clinical significance of antibodies and selection of units prior to issue

SYSTEM	ANTIBODY SPECIFICITY	CLINICAL SIGNIFICANCE	RECOMMENDATION
ABO	Anti-A_1	Rarely	Group A, D matched, IAT crossmatch compatible at $37^{\circ}C$ *
Rh	Anti-D, -C, -c, -E, -e (active by IAT)	Yes	Antigen negative (compatible by IAT at $37^{\circ}C$)
	Anti-C^w	Rarely	C negative, D matched, IAT crossmatch compatible at $37^{\circ}C$
Kell	Anti-K, -k	Yes	Antigen negative (compatible by IAT at $37^{\circ}C$)
	Anti-Kp^a	Rarely	ABO & D matched, IAT crossmatch compatible at $37^{\circ}C$ *
Kidd	Anti-Jk^a, -Jk^b	Yes	Antigen negative (compatible by IAT at $37^{\circ}C$)
MNS	Anti-M (active at $37^{\circ}C$)	Sometimes	Antigen negative (compatible by IAT at $37^{\circ}C$)
	Anti-M (not active at $37^{\circ}C$)	Rarely	ABO & D matched, IAT crossmatch compatible at $37^{\circ}C$ *
	Anti-N	Rarely	ABO & D matched, IAT crossmatch compatible at $37^{\circ}C$ *
	Anti-S, -s, -U	Yes	Antigen negative (compatible by IAT at $37^{\circ}C$)
Duffy	Anti-Fy^a, -Fy^b	Yes	Antigen negative (compatible by IAT at $37^{\circ}C$)
P	Anti-P_1	Rarely	ABO & D matched, IAT crossmatch compatible at $37^{\circ}C$ *
Lewis	Anti-Le^a, -Le^b, and -Le^{a+b}	Rarely / No	ABO & D matched, IAT crossmatch compatible at $37^{\circ}C$ *
Lutheran	Anti-Lu^a	Rarely	ABO & D matched, IAT crossmatch compatible at $37^{\circ}C$ *
Diego	Anti-Wr^a	Rarely	ABO & D matched, IAT crossmatch compatible at $37^{\circ}C$ *
H	Anti-HI (in A_1 and A_1B people)	No	ABO & D matched, IAT crossmatch compatible at $37^{\circ}C$ *
All others	Reactive by IAT at $37^{\circ}C$	Variable	Seek advice from Blood Centre

* Select blood that is of the same ABO and D type as the patient; specifically selected antigen negative blood is NOT required.
NOTE: The above guidance is also suitable for patients undergoing hypothermia during surgery

ADDITIONAL TRANSFUSION REQUIREMENTS

As well as the requirements of pre-transfusion testing described above, it is important to identify and make available any specific transfusion requirements for the patient, such as the need for fresh blood (for a neonate), CMV- products, etc.

VISUAL INSPECTION OF RED CELL UNITS

Before any unit is issued it should be checked to ensure that there is no:
- Leakage from the ports or seams of the blood bag
- Evidence of haemolysis in the plasma or at the interface between the red cells and plasma
- Discoloration of the red cells
- Presence of clots

If any of these are present, the unit should not be used for transfusion and should be returned to the Blood Centre with accompanying documentation.

RETENTION OF RECORDS

It is necessary to keep all laboratory worksheet, records, etc., for 30 years (see the section Sources of Additional Information for reference details and Section 15: Quality, for further information).

QUESTIONS - SECTION 8

1. What pre-transfusion laboratory procedures are recommended?

2. What laboratory procedures should (in preference) be performed prior to an emergency transfusion?

3. Explain the principles of the 'type and screen' procedure.

4. What is MSBOS and why is it used?

5. How long should crossmatch worksheets be kept prior to disposal?

6. What is an 'immediate spin' crossmatch and what is it primarily designed to detect?

7. What is 'electronic issue'?

8. Which blood group antibody specificities, detected prior to a crossmatch in a patient's serum/plasma requires the selection of antigen negative blood?

9. Which antibody specificities are rarely clinically significant?

10. The visible inspection of blood donations prior to issue from the laboratory should ensure what?

SECTION 9

TRANSFUSION REACTIONS

There are a number of reasons why a patient may have a reaction to a transfusion, the effects of which can vary greatly. Immune related reactions, involving an antigen-antibody reaction, can range from mild urticaria (an allergic reaction) that rarely needs treatment, through febrile reactions, involving shivering and fever, caused invariably by antibodies to white cells, to haemolytic reactions resulting from the destruction of transfused red cells.

HAZARDS OF TRANSFUSION

A hazard has been defined as 'any unfavourable event occurring in a patient during or following the transfusion of blood or a blood product'. There are theoretically numerous potentially unfavourable effects of transfusion, which can be categorised in a variety of different ways, based on different criteria. The hazards that are of specific interest to hospital laboratory transfusion scientists involve mainly those caused by immune (antigen-antibody) reactions. These may involve reactions to red cells, white cells, platelets or plasma, as well as allergic reactions. These immune reactions are a result of the recipient having a pre-formed antibody against an antigen that is subsequently transfused to the patient.

In the case of a reaction to red cells, because of the routine use of pre-transfusion *in vitro* testing regimes, any such hazard occurring should have been detected and could therefore be the result of an operational error (technical, clerical, etc.). With immune reactions involving white cells, platelets or plasma, prior knowledge of the presence of an antibody capable of causing a reaction is generally unknown since there are no pre-transfusion tests routinely used to detect them. In the case of antibodies to white cells, platelets and plasma, it is only when a reaction occurs in a patient and is investigated that antigen-negative material is considered and/or selected for subsequent transfusion.

Other potential hazards more specifically related to the products themselves, are for example bacterial contamination and disease transmission involving hepatitis, HIV, etc. In addition, there are a variety of potentially hazardous effects seen during or following a transfusion which are mainly related either to the transfusion procedure itself (e.g. air embolism) or are problems associated with the transfusion of specific patient groups (e.g. citrate toxicity, potassium toxicity).

SERIOUS HAZARDS OF TRANSFUSION (SHOT) SCHEME

Concerns regarding the incidence of errors and subsequent problems involving transfusions resulted in the formation in 1996 of the 'Serious Hazards of Transfusion' (SHOT) scheme. This national UK scheme monitors via a voluntary registration and confidential reporting process, all hazards identified to be associated with transfusion. The scheme covers the hazards associated with the transfusion of both blood components manufactured at blood centres as well as fractionated plasma products. The reporting system used is dependent upon the nature of the identified adverse event. Cases of bacterial contamination and post-transfusion infectious disease hazards are reported via the local Blood Centre who supplied the product. Whereas transfusion errors and other associated complications are reported directly to the SHOT scheme, all of which form the basis of a published annual report (see Sources of Additional information for further reference details).

The SHOT system has identified that the majority of problems associated with transfusion are currently categorised into:

- Incorrect blood component transfused (IBCT)
- Immune complications of transfusion;
  - Acute transfusion reactions (ATR)
  - Haemolytic transfusion reactions (HTR/DHTR)
  - Post transfusion purpura (PTP)
  - Transfusion-related acute lung injury (TRALI)
- Transfusion associated graft-versus-host-disease (TA-GvHD)
- Transfusion transmitted infections (TTI)

Also included are the following separate reporting categories of:

- Inappropriate/ unnecessary transfusions
- Handling & storage errors
- Near miss events
- Transfusion associated circulatory overload (TACO)
- Anti-D administration

Since the SHOT scheme was introduced it has identified a number of deaths that could be attributed directly to the transfusion event. The scheme has consistently identified that many of the laboratory-based errors are transcription errors or transposition of samples. Each annual SHOT report makes recommendations related to improving the safety of transfusions. A guideline document has also been published on 'the administration of blood and blood components and the management of transfused patients' (see Sources of Additional Information for reference details).

BLOOD SAFETY AND QUALITY REGULATIONS (BSQR) 2005 AND SABRE

On 8th February 2005 the new EU law concerning blood safety came into effect. A grace period to introduce the changes was granted but after 8th November 2005 the law became active. Changes to hospital blood banks governing aspects of quality, tracking all stages of donated blood from donor to recipient and back again, cold chain storage and the training of all staff are now mandatory. The blood bank can no longer change any blood product other than thawing FFP. If they wish to do so they must apply to the regulatory body for a producer's licence.

The regulatory body appointed by the government is the Medicines and Healthcare products Regulatory Agency (MHRA). All hospital blood banks have to register and re-register, giving details of how they fulfil the changes in the law. A new on-line reporting system, the Serious Adverse Blood Reactions and Events (SABRE) has been introduced, which is in addition to the paper SHOT reporting system, although SHOT data will largely be collected using the SABRE system - apart from Transfusion Transmitted Infection (TTI) returns. Participants are encouraged to report all events, including 'near misses', using this system. Any reports other than serious adverse reactions and events are highlighted for the attention of SHOT and the MHRA divert them. The reader is advised to be conversant with how both of these systems operate and to have knowledge of the content of the latest annual SHOT report (see Sources of Additional Information for reference details).

INCORRECT COMPONENT TRANSFUSED

This has been defined as 'the transfusion of a patient with a blood component, which does not meet the appropriate requirements or which was intended for another patient'. Studies, including the SHOT reports, have identified that many of these problems result from clerical errors. The transfusion of an incorrect blood component is invariably associated with a procedural failure and can be identified to be associated with the following areas:

- Prescription, sampling and requesting.
- Transfusion Laboratory :
    - Transposition of samples
    - Failure to consult/heed historical records
    - Technical error of grouping, screening or crossmatching
    - Selection/use of an inappropriate component
    - Incorrect labelling of component and/or issue voucher
- Collection (of incorrect component) and administration (failure of bedside checking process).
- Supply of incorrect material by the Blood Centre

The clerical errors are related to patient identification, blood sample labelling and/or procedural errors involving the collection of the units of blood from the hospital blood bank and its subsequent administration. It is important to follow local procedures for identifying patients, labelling samples and handling those samples in the laboratory. These are without exception avoidable errors and their occurrence has placed an even greater emphasis on the 'bedside check' in the final, vital step in preventing mis-transfusion. These procedures are increasingly being formalised and written into Standard Operating Procedures (SOPs) as well as being subject to audit and review by Hospital Transfusion Committees.

RED CELL INCOMPATIBILITY

Haemolytic transfusion reactions, resulting from a red cell incompatibility, may be either immediate / acute (occurring within 24 hours of the transfusion event) or delayed (occurring over 24 hours after the transfusion event). Immediate reactions are usually caused by the patient's ABO antibodies destroying the transfused red cells intravascularly as a result of the wrong A or B blood group being transfused, whereas red cell destruction in delayed reactions is extravascular, usually within the spleen.

Major / minor incompatibility

1. Major incompatibility is the term used to describe a reaction between the recipient's antibody and the transfused (donor) red cells. This is the most important type of incompatibility.
2. Minor incompatibility is the term used to describe a reaction between transfused antibody (in the donor plasma) and the recipient's red cells.

A variety of effects are possible as a result of a major incompatibility, primarily related to the following factors:

- The amount (titre) of antibody present in the patient's circulation
- The type of antibody present, i.e. related to:
  - Avidity
  - Blood group specificity
  - Immunoglobulin type (and sub-type)
  - Complement activating ability
- The amount of red cells transfused (smaller volumes are removed more rapidly)

Therefore, depending upon the variability of the above circumstances, *in vivo* red cell destruction can be demonstrated to result in either intravascular and/or extravascular red cell destruction.

Immediate (acute) Haemolytic Reactions

This type of reaction involves intravascular haemolysis, i.e. the rupture and breakdown of red cells in the blood stream by complement activation, resulting in the release of haemoglobin into the plasma. This occurs as a result of the action of potent complement fixing antibodies present in the patient's plasma at the time of the transfusion, together with the infusion of relatively small volumes of red cells which are positive for the corresponding antigen. This results in the activation and binding of complement components, the rupture of the red cells in the circulation (haemolysis) and an immediate reaction (see Section 2: Antibody Mediated Red Cell Destruction).

The major cause of immediate transfusion reactions and death from transfusion is due to transfusing the wrong patient (i.e. with blood intended for someone else) who is of a different ABO group. If this type of incident occurs, it is essential to check the records and labels of the other units which were cross-matched at the same time as the patient who has had the reaction, since the samples from two (or more) patients may have become mixed-up. This event could result in the blood intended for another patient also being wrongly labelled and transfused. Most of these accidents have been shown to occur through clerical / identification errors as a result of someone not having accurately followed the procedures for double-checking, designed to ensure that the correctly labelled blood is transfused into the right patient.

Acute transfusion reactions have also been reported with non-red cell products, i.e. fresh frozen plasma, white cells and platelets, which involve haemolytic, non-haemolytic, hypotensive and anaphylactic reactions.

Cytokines

The clinical effects of a haemolytic transfusion reaction are the result of the production of cytokines. Cytokines is the term used to describe a series of protein hormones that are involved in cell to cell communication. A number of these are generated during a haemolytic transfusion reaction, as a result of the complement activation and the generation of anaphylatoxins (C3a and C5a), that have potent inflammatory effects. ABO incompatibility rapidly involves stimulating the release of tumour necrosis factor (TNF), interleukins (principally IL-1 and IL-8) and monocyte chemo-attractant protein (MCP). By acting to release histamine from basophils and activation of T and B-lymphocytes, these molecules produce the effects of fever, hypotension and shock (see Section 2: Antibody Mediated Red Cell Destruction).

Delayed Haemolytic Reactions

Delayed transfusion reactions invariably occur in those patients who have received a primary antibody stimulation in the past, as a result of a transfusion or pregnancy. In the intervening time period, the antibody titre has fallen to a level at which it cannot be detected by routine pre-transfusion antibody screening and/or crossmatching tests. As a result of this, these patients may be transfused with red cells that (by chance) are antigen positive for the previously stimulated antibody specificity. Within a few days of the transfusion, a secondary (anamnestic) immune response develops which produces enough antibody to cause destruction of the now incompatible transfused red cells. This results in a fall in the patient's haemoglobin level, together with possible jaundice and fever.

It is important therefore to check any previous grouping and antibody screening results prior to transfusion (see Section 8: Pre-Transfusion Testing). This will identify if the patient has produced a clinically significant antibody specificity in the past (according to hospital patient records) but which is no longer detectable at the time of the current transfusion. If this is the case, antigen negative blood should be chosen, even though the clinically significant antibody is no longer detectable.

For a few days following the delayed reaction, the direct antiglobulin test (DAT) may be positive, with a 'mixed-field' appearance, as only the transfused red cells have antibody on their surface and therefore give a positive reaction; the patient's own red cells being negative. When most of the transfused red cells have been destroyed, free antibody appears in the serum. Anti-Jk^a is commonly associated with this type of reaction, though a number of other blood group antibody specificities have also been implicated.

The symptoms associated with a delayed transfusion reaction can vary and it may not be obvious that a delayed transfusion reaction has occurred. However, although not usually serious, when associated with the underlying disease, a delayed transfusion reaction may prove to be a fatal complication.

INVESTIGATION OF A SUSPECTED IMMEDIATE HAEMOLYTIC TRANSFUSION REACTION (HTR Acute)

The transfusion should be stopped immediately on identification of adverse symptoms and the following should be requested / sent immediately to the Blood Bank:

- The unit being transfused (together with the giving set)
- The remains of the units of blood and/or blood products transfused prior to the reaction being identified
- Fresh blood samples ('post-transfusion') from the patient
- Details of the reaction, e.g. the patient's symptoms, temperature, pulse, etc.

The symptoms of a haemolytic transfusion reaction vary, but may be dramatic and severe. Reported symptoms include fever, chills, a burning sensation at the site of the infusion, hypotension, chest-constriction, breathing problems, lower back/joint pains and shock. It is important that all identified symptoms are reported on the transfusion reaction investigation request form as this may indicate red cell / non-red cell involvement as well as an indication of the nature and severity of the reaction. This may give an early indication of the area of laboratory investigation required.

The basic procedures for the investigation of a suspected immediate (acute) HTR involve the following:

1. Check the patient's details against the units transfused and all other documentation to identify any clerical and/or labelling error. If a clerical/labelling error is identified, ensure that checks are performed to exclude the involvement of another patient.
2. Centrifuge the post-transfusion sample and examine the serum/plasma for haemolysis.
3. Perform ABO and D grouping and a DAT on the patient's pre-transfusion (laboratory stored) and post-transfusion blood samples as well as each of the units transfused; include those units transfused prior to the one suspected of causing the reaction.
4. Repeat the antibody screening tests on both pre- and post-transfusion patient blood samples and repeat cross-match both the pre- and post-transfusion samples with all units transfused.
5. The units of blood transfused should be checked for possible bacterial infection (if appropriate - related to the reported symptoms).
6. In addition, further tests may be performed on the patient as required, e.g. clotting screens if the patient is suffering from Disseminated Intravascular Coagulation (DIC). In the absence of any indication of red cell incompatibility and dependant upon the patient's symptoms (e.g. febrile), additional procedures including tests for white cell and/or platelet antibodies may be required on the patient's pre-transfusion sample.

If evidence of a transfusion reaction is found, senior scientific staff and the consultant haematologist should be informed immediately to decide what further action is necessary. This may include a review of existing procedures and the reporting of the incident to the MHRA via the SABRE on-line reporting scheme.

INVESTIGATION OF A SUSPECTED DELAYED HAEMOLYTIC TRANSFUSION REACTION

If a delayed reaction is suspected, a DAT on the post-transfusion sample should be performed, followed by repeating the antibody screening tests on the pre- and post-transfusion samples. If the DAT is positive (this will be 'mixed-field') and no free antibody is detected in the patient's serum/plasma samples, the antibody should be eluted from the red cells and identified. Once the antibody specificity has been identified, antigen negative blood should be selected for any further crossmatching. As above, senior staff should be consulted if there is serological evidence of a delayed reaction having occurred.

TRANSFUSION RELATED ACUTE LUNG INJURY (TRALI)

TRALI is defined as an acute reaction involving dyspnoea (difficult or laboured breathing) with hypoxia (oxygen deficiency) and may involve chills, fever and a non-productive cough. The condition is however characterised by bilateral pulmonary infiltrates (nodules on the lung) occurring during or within 24 hours of transfusion, with no other apparent cause.

The reaction is frequently severe, a proportion of which are fatal. The mechanism causing the condition is unknown, but is classically associated with the transfusion of (relatively small volumes) of high titre complement activating leucocyte (WBC) antibodies present in the donor's plasma. As such, any investigation of a suspected TRALI reaction should involve notification of the Blood Centre, which provided the product and the serological investigation of the donor(s) involved. Different antibody specificities (including Human Leucocyte Antigen - HLA) have been reported to be responsible, reactive against lymphocytes and granulocytes.

POST-TRANSFUSION PURPURA (PTP)

PTP is defined as thrombocytopenia arising normally 5-12 days following a transfusion of a red cell / platelet concentrate product, which is associated with the presence in the patient of antibodies directed against the human platelet antigen (HPA) systems.

The reaction is caused by the presence of a platelet specific antibody in a patient, which reacts with transfused antigen positive platelets. Different platelet antibody specificities have been implicated, though is usually anti-HPA-1a. The platelet specific antibody may be produced as a result of a previous transfusion but is most frequently produced by women as a result of immunisation via a previous pregnancy. The PTP condition may be severe and involve the destruction of the patient's own antigen negative platelets via an 'innocent bystander' mechanism.

Treatment involves the use of intra-venous immunoglobulin and any further transfusion support should normally involve the use of selected antigen-negative platelet donations.

TRANSFUSION-ASSOCIATED GRAFT-VERSUS-HOST-DISEASE (TA-GvHD)

TA-GvHD is defined as the development of the classic symptoms of fever, rash, liver dysfunction, diarrhoea and pancytopenia occurring 1-6 weeks following transfusion, without any other apparent cause. Skin/bone marrow biopsy and the appearance and/or presence of circulating donor lymphocytes usually support the diagnosis. This is a rare complication of transfusion associated with other underlying patient conditions (e.g. malignancies) and is caused by the transfusion of viable donor white cells. The condition is more likely to occur when the patient and donor share (by chance) an HLA haplotype. The condition has been shown to be reduced by the use of pre-transfusion gamma-irradiation of cellular components which is designed to inhibit the DNA replication of white cells (see also 'Guidelines on gamma-irradiation of blood components for the prevention of transfusion-associated graft-versus-host-disease', see Sources of Additional Information for reference details).

TRANSFUSION-TRANSMITTED INFECTIONS (TTI)

TTI are rare and differ from other complications in that the onset of symptoms related to the viral infection may occur from several weeks to years after the transfusion. In addition, any suspected transmission involves tracing and re-testing the donor(s) involved as well as the identification of any other recipients of the donor material who may be asymptomatic and only identified via the investigation. The investigation is obviously complicated by the fact that a suspected post-transfusion infection may have been acquired from another source. Subsequent identification of a viral marker in an implicated donor or the finding of a positive result in a subsequent donation from a donor can affirm transfusion as the probable source of infection. As a result, the Blood Service must be involved in any investigation of a possible TTI.

The risk of disease transmission by transfusion is initially reduced by the questioning of blood donors and the pre-donation screening out of 'high risk' donors based on national Donor Selection Guidelines. However, to reduce the incidence of TTI, the Blood Services perform mandatory microbiology testing of each donation for a number of infection markers. These are currently hepatitis B (HBV), hepatitis C (HCV), human immunodeficiency virus HIV (the infective agent for AIDS) and syphilis (see Section 13: Blood Donation Testing).

Bacterial Contamination

This is an uncommon hazard of transfusion, kept at a low incidence by the use of disposable plastic blood packs and sterile materials. However, the transfusion of even small amounts of infected blood is frequently fatal. If bacterial contamination does occur, it has been shown to be associated with either:

- Contamination during blood collection, due to the presence of (deep seated) bacteria (e.g. Pseudomonas species) in the donor's skin at the venepuncture site, which is not removed by the routine skin cleaning procedures used prior to donating. The bacteria enter the blood pack via a 'skin plug', which is the source of the infection.
- The donor has an asymptomatic low-grade bacteraemia at the time of donation (e.g. *Yersinia enterocolitica*).
- Bacterial contamination occurring during storage via an undetected 'pin-hole' leak in the blood pack, i.e. resulting from a blood bag manufacturing defect or due to inadequate (heat) sealing of bleed lines during processing.

Storage at 4°C does not remove the problem as some bacteria can grow rapidly in blood at low temperatures, producing bacterial pyrogenic material, i.e. bacterial lipopolysaccharides and storage of platelet concentrates at 22°C may enhance bacterial growth. The transfusion of infected blood results (to varying degrees) in symptoms of fever, hypotension and leucopenia, and may involve pain in the abdomen and extremities, with vomiting and bloody diarrhoea. The symptoms normally appear after a latent period of approximately 30 minutes and may follow the infusion of very small volumes of blood. Transfusion of bacterially infected blood often proves fatal (see Section 13: Blood Donation Testing).

SERIOUS HAZARDS OF TRANSFUSION - SUMMARY OF THE MAIN FEATURES OF ADVERSE EVENTS AND DIAGNOSTIC TESTS

(The table below is reproduced from the 'SHOT Annual Report 1997/98' with permission of The Serious Hazards of Transfusion Steering Group)

	PROBLEM	TYPICAL FEATURES	DIAGNOSTIC TESTS
1	a. Incorrect blood or component transfused: ABO incompatible	May be none - or major collapse as for 2.	Check identity and group of patient and unit (inc. Rh D). May have positive DAT.
	b. Incorrect blood or component transfused: ABO compatible	May be none. As for 2 if patient has atypical red cell alloantibodies.	Check identity and group of patient and unit (inc. Rh D). May have positive DAT.
2	Acute haemolytic transfusion reaction	Dyspnoea, chest pain, fever, chills, ↓ BP, ↓ urine output, DIC.	Haemoglobinaemia/uria, ↓ Hb, positive DAT, serological incompatibility, spherocytes in blood film.
	Anaphylaxis	↓BP, dyspnoea, ± bronchospasm, ± rash.	Occasionally severe IgA deficiency with anti-IgA.
3	Delayed haemolytic transfusion reaction	Unexplained fall in Hb, jaundice, dark urine.	Urobilinogen in urine, ↑ serum bilirubin, positive DAT, spherocytes, positive antibody screen.
4	Transfusion-associated graft-versus-host-disease (TA-GvHD)	Progression of fever, rash, ↑ liver enzymes, diarrhoea, pancytopenia (1-6 weeks post transfusion.	Skin biopsy, positive cytogenic or HLA analysis. DNA analysis (e.g. RFLP, minisatellite probes) to establish presence of third party lymphocytes.
5	Transfusion-related acute lung injury (TRALI)	Acute respiratory distress (non cardiogenic). Hypoxia, bilateral pulmonary infiltrates.	Anti-leucocyte antibodies in donor or recipient.
6	Post-transfusion purpura (PTP)	Immune-mediated thrombocytopenia arising 5-12 days post-transfusion.	HPA type patient, HPA antibodies (usually HPA-1a negative with anti-HPA-1a).
7	Reaction to a bacterially contaminated component	Rapid onset of circulatory collapse, fever.	REFER TO BLOOD CENTRE URGENTLY.
8	Post transfusion viral infection	Depends on virus, e.g. jaundice, malaise, rash. Weeks to months post transfusion.	REFER TO BLOOD CENTRE URGENTLY.
9	Other	Any other severe adverse reaction associated with transfusion of a blood component.	

QUESTIONS - SECTION 9

1. What is the major cause of severe immediate haemolytic transfusion reactions?

2. Explain the mechanism causing a delayed transfusion reaction to occur.

3. What is the most common error that results in a transfusion reaction?

4. TTI are reduced by what processes?

5. What is TRALI and what causes it?

6. What is PTP and what causes it?

7. What is TA-GvHD and what causes it?

8. Bacterial contamination of a blood donation can occur by what processes?

9. Identify the basic procedure for the investigation of a suspected immediate transfusion reaction.

10. Why is a positive DAT result 'mixed-field' in a delayed transfusion reaction?

ASSIGNMENT

From your Blood Bank records can you identify an incident of a reported transfusion reaction and if so, was the cause able to be identified?

SECTION 10

OTHER BLOOD GROUP SYSTEMS

Classically, a blood group system must include two or more antithetical antigens which are produced as a result of the action of a pair (or pairs) of allelic genes at a single independent genetic locus.

The ABO and Rh blood group systems have already been described in Sections 3 and 4 respectively. These are the two major blood group systems with regard to clinical significance. Although there are a total of 29 blood group systems currently recognised by the International Society for Blood Transfusion (ISBT), historically there are recognised to be nine 'major' blood group systems.

In addition, there have been described a large number of separate individual antigen-antibody specificities, which have been demonstrated to not be part of any of the known blood group systems. Some of these may, in the future, be found to have allelic gene (antithetical antigen) partners and would therefore be 'promoted' to the status of a blood group system.

As with the ABO and Rh blood group systems, the red cell antigens of the other blood group systems are the result of the action of specific structural genes resulting in the production of specific protein or carbohydrate structures within the red cell membrane.

BLOOD GROUP NOMENCLATURE

There is a bewildering variety of terminologies used for representing the large number of different blood group antigens, genes, phenotypes and genotypes. Although understandably difficult, the correct application of blood group terminology is however essential to ensure that information is accurately transmitted.

The terminology for antigens produced by allelic genes has changed with time. Initially these were represented and written by the use of different capital letters, e.g. A and B, M and N, then capital and small script letters, e.g. S and s, K and k, etc., followed by superscript letters, e.g. Fy^a and Fy^b, Jk^a and Jk^b, etc., and most recently by the use of numbers, e.g. Sc1 and Sc2, etc. It is convention to identify phenotype designations using positive and negative symbols, e.g. a red cell shown to have the D antigen as D+, etc., some of which should be enclosed by brackets and none of the letters should be superscript, e.g. Le(a+b-), Fy(a-b+), etc. When the numerical nomenclature is used, the absence of an antigen is identified by a minus symbol and antigen presence simply by the use of the number, e.g. Sc: -1,2. Genes (representing the presence of an antigen) are denoted in text by the use of italics.

Interpretation of data and the mis-use of nomenclature

It is incorrect to assume that a person who has been grouped with a single antibody specificity and found negative is therefore positive for the antithetical antigen, e.g. red cells that have been grouped using only anti-K and found to be negative cannot be inferred to be k+. Similarly, only when someone has been grouped with antisera defining both antigens can a genotype be inferred. Grouping a person's red cells, to establish that they are antigen-negative is commonly used to help confirm the specificity of an antibody. The International Society of Blood Transfusion (ISBT) has implemented a numerical terminology for the different blood groups systems, which is intended for computer use. Each blood group system is allocated a three-digit number (see table below) followed by a second three-digit number to represent each antigen within that system, e.g. the B antigen is represented as 001002.

Examples of the nomenclature used in the nine 'major' blood group systems

BLOOD GROUP	ISBT NUMBER	MAJOR ANTIGEN NAMES	ANTIGEN / PHENOTYPE DESIGNATION
ABO	001	A B	A A_1 A_2 B O AB A_1B A_2B
Rh	004	C c D E e	C+ C- c+ c- D+ D- E+ E- e+ e- i.e. as C+c-D+E-e+
MNS	002	M N S s	M+ M- N+ N- S+ S- s+ s- i.e. as M+N+S+s-
P	003	P_1 P	P_1 and P_2 i.e. as P_1+ and P_1-
Kell	006	K k Kp^a Kp^b Js^a Js^b	K+ K- k+ k- i.e. as K+k+ Kp(a-b+) Js(a-b+)
Duffy	008	Fy^a Fy^b	Fy(a+) Fy(a-) Fy(b+) Fy(b-) i.e. as Fy(a+b+)
Kidd	009	Jk^a Jk^b	Jk(a+) Jk(a-) Jk(b+) Jk(b-) i.e. as Jk(a+b+)
Lewis	007	Le^a Le^b	Le(a+) Le(a-) Le(b+) Le(b-) i.e. as Le(a-b-)
Lutheran	005	Lu^a Lu^b	Lu(a+) Lu(a-) Lu(b+) Lu(b-) i.e. as Lu(a-b+)

BLOOD GROUP FREQUENCIES

Blood group frequencies may vary greatly between different races and therefore phenotypes rarely encountered in one particular race may be extremely common in another. All frequencies quoted in this section are approximate and for UK Whites, unless otherwise stated. The incidence of a particular antigen or more accurately, its absence, in the UK population relates directly to the ease or difficulty with which antigen-negative and therefore compatible units of blood are able to be made available for a patient with the particular antibody specificity. Blood group frequencies are therefore practically important.

The absence of both alleles at a particular blood group locus (due to a variety of genetic backgrounds) is termed a "minus-minus" or "null" phenotype and is rare in all of the major blood group systems described within this section, with the exception of Lewis. Some minus-minus phenotype people may be stimulated by transfusion or pregnancy to produce an antibody which is positive with all red cell samples except those from other very rare examples of the minus-minus phenotype.

THE MNS BLOOD GROUP SYSTEM

The allelic genes *MN* and *Ss* have been shown to be very closely linked, i.e. the genes are very close together on the same chromosome. These two pairs of alleles therefore form a single blood group system, called 'MNS'. The linkage between the *MN* and *Ss* genes was identified from MN and Ss grouping a large number of people. This showed the S antigen and therefore the *S* gene is more commonly seen in M+ than in M- people, i.e. the *S* gene is genetically linked to the *M* gene. This genetic linkage results in frequency variations, which would not be seen if the *MN* and *Ss* genes were unlinked (inherited independently), e.g. M+N-S+ frequency is 20% whereas M-N+S+ frequency is 6%. Although a single blood group system, it is easier and more relevant practically, to deal with MN and Ss separately.

MN

M and N antigen production is coded for by a single pair of co-dominant genes, resulting in the production of three common phenotypes:

| RED CELL REACTIONS WITH | | PHENOTYPE | GENOTYPE | APPROX. UK FREQUENCY |
Anti-M	Anti-N			
+	-	M+ N-	*MM*	28%
+	+	M+ N+	*MN*	50%
-	+	M- N+	*NN*	22%

The MN antigens are defined by a difference in two amino-acids at positions 1 and 5 of a 131 amino-acid long red cell membrane spanning (structural) protein known as glycophorin A (GPA). GPA contributes to the net negative charge of the red cell membrane, since it is the most abundant sialoglycoprotein, i.e. over 200,000 copies per red cell. Being defined by terminal amino-acids, the M and N antigens are destroyed by protease enzyme treatment, which removes glycoprotein from the red cell membrane (see Section 2: Antigen - Antibody Reactions). As a result, anti-M and anti-N antibodies do not work by routine enzyme (papain) techniques.

Anti-M and anti-N antibodies have occasionally been described as having been produced as a result of stimulation by environmental factors as "naturally occurring" antibodies. More usually however, they are stimulated as a result of red cell immunisation by transfusion or rarely pregnancy. Both antibodies usually work by the saline agglutination technique and at temperatures up to 20°C, though some examples, especially anti-M, may also react up to 37°C. Although this may suggest that anti-M and anti-N antibodies are mainly IgM immunoglobulin, many are reported to be either IgG only or to contain an IgG component. The antibodies do not readily activate complement.

Although involvement of both antibodies has been described in transfusion reaction and HDFN events, such occurrences are very rare and both anti-M and anti-N antibodies are normally considered to have little clinical significance. The antibody reactivity at 37°C is a criterion used to identify if antigen negative blood should be used for crossmatching, if the anti-M or anti-N is non-reactive by IAT at 37°C, blood which is crossmatch compatible only can be used for transfusion. However, if the anti-M or anti-N is reactive by IAT at 37°C, antigen negative blood should be used for crossmatching (see Section 8: Pre-Transfusion Testing).

Ss

S and s antigen production is coded for by a single pair of co-dominant genes, resulting in the production of three common phenotypes:

RED CELL REACTIONS WITH		PHENOTYPE	GENOTYPE	APPROX. UK FREQUENCY
Anti-S	Anti-s			
+	-	S+ s-	SS	11%
+	+	S+ s+	Ss	44%
-	+	S- s+	ss	45%

The Ss antigens are defined by a single amino-acid substitution at position 29 of a 72 amino-acid long red cell membrane spanning structural protein known as glycophorin B (GPB). As such, like the MN antigens, the Ss antigens are also affected by protease enzyme activity. As a result, anti-S antibodies are not detectable by routine enzyme (e.g. papain) techniques, whilst the reactivity of examples of examples of anti-s is variable, dependant upon the technique and/or enzyme employed.

Although the Ss antigens are almost always present in UK Whites (see above chart), the phenotype S-s- is seen in Black populations. The presence of S and/or s is associated with a high frequency protease resistant antigen called U. People who are S-s- may be either U- or U+, whereas U- red cells are always S-s-.

Anti-S and anti-s are usually IgG immune antibodies and are both clinically significant, having been implicated in transfusion reactions and occasionally severe or fatal HDFN. Although some examples of anti-s have been described to be optimally active at 20°C, both antibody specificities are capable of activating complement and are usually reactive at 37°C by AHG techniques. As such, antigen negative blood should be selected for crossmatching when either of these antibody specificities are present in the patient's serum/plasma.

Anti-U antibodies, produced by people of the rare U negative phenotype, are immune stimulated normally non-complement fixing IgG antibodies, capable of causing severe transfusion reactions and severe/fatal HDFN. Note: U negative phenotype red cells are always S-s-, whereas S-s- phenotype red cells may be either U+ or U-.

THE P BLOOD GROUP SYSTEM

There are two common phenotypes in the P blood group system, P$_1$ (frequency 75%) and P$_2$ (frequency 25%) produced by the presence or absence of the P$_1$ antigen. The antigen is glycolipid and the P blood group genetic locus is on chromosome number 22. The ISBT designation for this blood group system is P1.

Group P$_2$ people can produce anti-P$_1$ when stimulated by P$_1$ positive red cells. Anti-P$_1$ is a relatively commonly occurring though normally weakly reacting antibody, which has been reported to be either immune or more commonly 'naturally occurring', only rarely having been described as having been stimulated by transfusion. Examples of anti-P$_1$ are usually IgM, do not normally activate complement and invariably react best at temperatures up to 20°C. As such, these antibodies are normally detected by saline techniques and may possibly be reactive in an ABO reverse group and are not clinically significant. On rare occasions examples of anti-P$_1$ may react up to 37°C, by AHG techniques; such examples may then be clinically significant. Anti- P$_1$ has not been reported as being implicated in causing HDFN.

The very rare 'minus-minus' phenotype of the P system, called "pp" or Tj(a-), which does not express either the P or P_1 antigens, commonly produces an antibody capable of reacting at $37^{\circ}C$ with all P positive (i.e. groups P_1 and P_2) red cells. This antibody is called anti-Tj^a (or anti-$P+P_1+P^k$) and is clinically significant.

THE KELL BLOOD GROUP SYSTEM

Although there are many antigens produced as a result of the complex genetics of this blood group system, there are two major co-dominant allelic genes at the Kell genetic locus producing two antithetical antigens (which are commonly encountered in blood group serology), the K (Kell) and the k (Cellano) antigens.

RED CELL REACTIONS WITH		PHENOTYPE	GENOTYPE	APPROX. UK FREQUENCY
Anti-K	Anti-k			
+	-	K+ k-	KK	0.2%
+	+	K+ k+	Kk	8.8%
-	+	K- k+	kk	91.0%

The Kell blood group system antigens are defined by a single amino-acid difference within a 732 amino acid long trans-membrane glycoprotein, believed to have an endopeptidase hormone function. All Kell (and para-Kell) antigens are destroyed by the chemical dithiothreitol (DTT) at a concentration of 100-200mM (DTT is used to break down and inactivate IgM immunoglobulin molecules). A mixture of 100mM DTT and 0.1% papain ('ZZAP' solution) also inactivates all Kell antigens (ZZAP solution is used during auto-adsorption procedures to remove autoantibody in the investigation of a positive DAT).

The K antigen is the most immunogenic outside the ABO and Rh blood group systems and as such anti-K is a relatively commonly produced antibody. It is commonly found as a single specificity in a patient's sample, but is also frequently found in combination with other antibody specificities. Anti-K and anti-k are invariably IgG immune antibodies, reacting best at $37^{\circ}C$ by AHG and enzyme techniques. The antibodies may activate complement and are clinically significant, having been implicated in both transfusion reactions and HDFN (occasionally severely or fatally). The k antigen appears to be a poor immunogen and together with the fact that only 0.2% of the population is the genotype KK, who are the only people able to produce anti-k when immunised, results in anti-k being a very rare antibody.

The presence of either antibody specificity in a patient's blood sample requires the selection of antigen negative blood for crossmatching prior to transfusion. Although anti-K is a relatively commonly encountered specificity, the identification of antigen negative units is a simple matter since approximately 9 out of 10 units will be K-negative (genotype kk). The finding of antigen negative blood for a patient with anti-k is however difficult since the frequency of k-negative (genotype KK) is only approximately 1 in 500.

Other Kell system antigens

Approximately 25 Kell system alleles and Kell related ('para-Kell') genes have been described, together with at least two phenotypic associations with other independent genetic loci (Kx and Gerbich). This makes the Kell blood group system second only to Rh in its complexity.

Kp^a and Kp^b

The Kp^a antigen is found in approximately 2% of the population, whereas Kp^b is very common with ~99.9% of the population being positive for this antigen. Both antibodies are rare. Anti-Kp^a is rarely clinically significant. Both antibodies react by IAT at 37°C.

Js^a and Js^b

The Js^a antigen is very rare in Whites, being found in <0.1% of people, whereas approximately 20% of Blacks are Js(a+). The Js^b antigen on the other hand is very common, being present in >99.9% of Whites and 98.9% of Blacks. Both antibodies are very rare, are clinically significant and react by IAT at 37°C.

The Kell system has a rare 'minus-minus' phenotype, i.e. K-k- Kp(a-b-) Js(a-b-), called K_o that is caused by the homozygous presence of a recessive gene (K^o) at the Kell locus resulting in the red cells lacking all Kell and para-Kell antigens. Immunised K_o patients may produce a single specificity antibody (anti-K_u) which reacts with all red cells except other examples of K_o.

THE DUFFY BLOOD GROUP SYSTEM

The two common red cell antigens of the Duffy blood group system, Fy^a and Fy^b, are produced as a result of the action of a pair of co-dominant allelic genes.

RED CELL REACTIONS WITH		PHENOTYPE	GENOTYPE	APPROX. UK FREQUENCY
Anti-Fy^a	Anti-Fy^b			
+	-	Fy(a+b-)	Fy^aFy^a	20%
+	+	Fy(a+b+)	Fy^aFy^b	47%
-	+	Fy(a-b+)	Fy^bFy^b	33%

Antigens of the Duffy system are defined within a protein that spans the red cell membrane nine times and functions as the red cell chemokine receptor that binds chemotactic and pro-inflammatory soluble peptides. The Fy^a and Fy^b antigens are the result of a single amino acid substitution within this 338 amino acid long protein. The Fy^a and Fy^b antigens are destroyed by treatment with proteolytic enzymes and therefore anti-Fy^a and anti-Fy^b are not reactive by enzyme (papain) techniques.

Anti-Fy^a and anti-Fy^b are IgG, active at 37°C by AHG techniques. Anti-Fy^a is a common antibody, estimated to be only three times less frequently produced than anti-K. Although occasionally stimulated by pregnancy, the majority of examples of anti-Fy^a are stimulated by transfusion. Anti-Fy^b is a relatively rare antibody. Examples of anti-Fy^a and anti-Fy^b frequently occur within a mixture of other antibody specificities (typically Rh). Both antibody specificities are clinically significant, having caused both transfusion reactions and HDFN. Antigen negative donations should be selected for crossmatching for patients with Duffy antibodies.

The Duffy blood group system antigen frequencies show marked variation between different populations. The Fy(a-b-) red cell ('minus-minus') phenotype is very rare in Whites but is found in as many as 76% of some Black populations in West Africa and as high as 97% in Central Africa. Red cells of the phenotype Fy(a-b-) have been shown to be resistant to invasion by the malarial parasite *Plasmodium vivax* (*in vivo*). It is therefore an advantage for Black Africans to lack Duffy red cell antigens.

THE KIDD BLOOD GROUP SYSTEM

There are two common red cell antigens of the Kidd blood group system, Jk^a and Jk^b, produced as a result of the action of a pair of co-dominant allelic genes.

RED CELL REACTIONS WITH		PHENOTYPE	GENOTYPE	APPROX. UK FREQUENCY
Anti-Jk^a	Anti-Jk^b			
+	-	Jk(a+b-)	Jk^aJk^a	26%
+	+	Jk(a+b+)	Jk^aJk^b	50%
-	+	Jk(a-b+)	Jk^bJk^b	24%

The Jk^a and Jk^b antigen reactivity provides a good example of 'dosage effect'. Dosage effect occurs as a result of the production of more antigen by the homozygote genotype than the heterozygote genotype, therefore more Jk^a antigen is present on Jk(a+b-) red cells than on Jk(a+b+) red cells. The respective antibody therefore reacts stronger against the homozygote person's red cells compared with red cells from the heterozygote. This effect can occasionally be seen in other blood groups. This is significant in antibody detection and crossmatching techniques (see Section 7: Antibody Detection and Identification) and is especially important with Kidd specificity antibodies, which have been reported to show marked variability in titre and strength of reaction between different examples.

The majority of anti-Jk^a and anti-Jk^b antibodies are reported to be immune IgG complement activating antibodies, stimulated by transfusion and/or pregnancy. The antibodies are active at $37^{\circ}C$ and are best detected by the AHG technique, but may also be detected by enzyme techniques. Both specificities are clinically significant having been implicated in transfusion reactions and are frequently associated with delayed transfusion reactions that are sometimes severe, but only rarely are associated with causing HDFN even though Kidd antigens are well developed at birth. Antigen negative red cells should be selected for crossmatching for a patient who has a Kidd specificity antibody.

THE LEWIS BLOOD GROUP SYSTEM

Lewis is unique among the major blood group systems described within this section in that the antigens are not red cell produced but are glycolipid plasma secretions, which are adsorbed onto the red cell membrane from the plasma.

The presence of the Lewis antigens, Le^a and Le^b, on the red cells of a person depends on the presence or absence of a number of genes at three different genetic loci, i.e. the Lewis gene (Le), the H gene and the genes enabling the H antigen to be secreted (the secretor genes, Se and se). The genotype backgrounds which result in the Lewis blood group antigens being present on the red cells is therefore very complex.

NOTE: The lack of clinical significance associated with Lewis antibodies would normally indicate that only a limited amount of information is provided in this book about this blood group system. However the complex nature of the underlying genetics and unusual phenotype expression of the Lewis system antigens frequently results in confusion. Although standard texts should be consulted, the following brief summary is provided to help the student:

The *Le* gene product is a transferase enzyme that catalyses the transfer of the carbohydrate L-fucose onto a sub-terminal N-acetyl-D-glucosamine carbohydrate, which is present in either of two possible substrates, 'precursor substance' and secreted H substance (see diagram below). The 'preferred' substrate if present is secreted H substance, which is only available when an individual has both the *H* and *Se* genes (i.e. people who are 'non-Bombay secretors'). If secreted, H substance is converted by the action of the *Le* gene enzyme product into the Le^b antigen. In the absence of secreted H substance, either because of the presence of the genotypes *hh* (Bombay group) and/or *sese* (non-secretors) the enzyme product of the *Le* gene acts on the precursor substance of H, which it converts into the Le^a antigen. Therefore, by acting on either of two different substrates, the enzyme produced by a single *Le* gene is capable of producing either Le^a or Le^b antigen product. If no *Le* gene is present, irrespective of the presence / absence of *H* and/or *Se* genes, neither of the antigens are produced and the person is therefore phenotype Le(a-b-). If produced, the Le^a or Le^b antigen material is subsequently adsorbed onto the red cells. Under normal circumstances therefore the Le^a and Le^b antigens are not produced at the same time and therefore the Le(a+b+) phenotype is not seen.

As a result of this complex genetic background, the production of the red cell Le^a and Le^b antigens can be summarised as follows:

- The red cell phenotype Le(a+b-) occurs in people who are ABH non-secretors.
- The red cell phenotype Le(a-b+) occurs in people who are ABH secretors.
- The red cell phenotype Le(a-b-) occurs in people who lack a Lewis gene and are therefore the genotype *lele*. Le(a-b-) people can therefore be either secretors or non-secretors.

This complex genetic background means that unlike the majority of other blood group systems, the heterozygote phenotype Le(a+b+) is not normally produced, whereas the 'minus-minus' phenotype Le(a-b-) is more commonly seen. Such individuals are capable of producing the antibody anti-Le^a+Le^b. In addition, Lewis antigens are not present at birth, unlike the antigens of the other major blood group systems, but develop during the first 15 months of life.

RED CELL REACTIONS WITH		PHENOTYPE	GENOTYPE *	APPROX. UK FREQUENCY
Anti-Le^a	Anti-Le^b			
+	-	Le(a+b-)	*H Le sese*	22%
-	+	Le(a-b+)	*H Le Se*	72%
-	-	Le(a-b-)	*H lele*	6%

* See text for explanation

Due to the fact that the antigens are adsorbed onto the red cells from the plasma in variable amounts, it is occasionally possible for the Lewis phenotype of a person to become weaker or even temporarily 'disappear', changing a person's red cell phenotype from say Le(a-b+) to Le(a-b-). This may be most frequently seen during pregnancy or in patients who are on steroid therapy. During these periods it is also possible for the person to transiently produce an anti-Le^b antibody.

Anti-Le^a and anti-Le^b antibody specificities regularly appear to be 'naturally occurring'. The antibodies may be detected as single specificities or produced together, i.e. as anti-Le^a+Le^b in people who are phenotype Le(a-b-). They are usually IgM, and even if IgG do not cause HDFN since fetal red cells are Le(a-b-). Both antibodies react by saline techniques normally up to 20°C, but some antibodies may react at 37°C and may be active by AHG techniques. Due to the fact that the Le^a and Le^b antigens are present as non-red cell secreted antigens, both anti-Le^a and anti-Le^b are capable of being inhibited by appropriate plasma, i.e. from an ABH non-secretor and secretor respectively.

Lewis antibodies rarely cause transfusion reactions and are therefore of limited clinical significance. Some antibody examples however may activate complement and cause haemolysis of test red cells *in vitro* (in freshly taken clotted blood samples). Patients with anti-Le^a, -Le^b or -Le^a+Le^b do not require antigen negative blood for crossmatching (see Section 8: Pre-Transfusion Testing).

Anti-Le^b antibodies have been classified as either anti-Le^{bH}, which preferentially react *in vitro* with red cells that have a high H antigen level (e.g. with Le(b+) group O and A$_2$), or as anti-Le^{bL} that agglutinate Le(b+) red cells *in vitro* irrespective of ABO group.

Basic chemical structural relationship between H and Lewis blood group antigens

PRECURSOR SUBSTANCE (PS): X -- Gal -- GlcNAc -- Gal

H SUBSTANCE:

X -- Gal -- GlcNAc -- Gal
|
Fuc

Le^a SUBSTANCE (i.e. converted PS):

X -- Gal -- GlcNAc – Gal
|
Fuc

Le^b SUBSTANCE (i.e. converted H):

X -- Gal -- GlcNAc -- Gal
| |
Fuc   Fuc

Abbreviations used for structures in the above diagrams:

X   : represents a long (branched) carbohydrate chain attached to protein (secreted glycoprotein).
GalNAc   : N-acetyl-D-galactosamine
GlcNAc   : N-acetyl-D-glucosamine
Fuc   : L-fucose
Gal   : D-galactose

THE LUTHERAN BLOOD GROUP SYSTEM

There are two major antigens of the Lutheran blood group system, one of which is rare (Lu^a) and the other very common (Lu^b), which are produced as a result of the action of a pair of co-dominant allelic genes.

RED CELL REACTIONS WITH		PHENOTYPE	GENOTYPE	APPROX. UK FREQUENCY
Anti-Lu^a	Anti-Lu^b			
+	-	Lu(a+b-)	*Lu^{a}Lu^a*	0.1%
+	+	Lu(a+b+)	*Lu^{a}Lu^b*	7.5%
-	+	Lu(a-b+)	*Lu^{b}Lu^b*	92.4%

Note: An Lu(a+) frequency of approximately 8% has been described in Europeans, Africans and North Americans, but is very rare or absent from all other populations studied.

In addition, there are three further pairs of alleles / antigens and 10 other high frequency antigens which have been described that are part of the Lutheran blood group system. In 1991, the Auberger antigens (Au^a and Au^b) were also shown to be part of the Lutheran blood group system.

Lutheran antigens are only weakly expressed on cord red cells. Lutheran antigens are destroyed by treatment of the red cells with trypsin or chymotrypsin; papain however has little if any effect. The Lutheran glycoprotein is believed to play a role in cell adhesion, probably during erythropoesis and is therefore thought to have little or no function in mature red cells. The Lutheran system has an Lu(a-b-) 'minus-minus' red cell phenotype (Lu$_{null}$), which can result either from either a recessive or a dominant genetic background. The frequency of the Lu$_{null}$ phenotype in the UK is estimated to be approximately 0.02%.

Anti-Lu^a and anti-Lu^b are both rarely produced and then are usually found in the serum/plasma of a person who has also produced antibodies to other blood group antigen specificities. Anti-Lu^a antibodies are usually IgM, active by saline techniques up to 20°C (rarely to 37°C), whereas anti-Lu^b antibodies are normally IgG, active by AHG techniques at 37°C. Anti-Lu^b antibodies show variable clinical significance whereas anti-Lu^a antibodies are rarely clinically significant.

THE Ii ANTIGENS AND ANTIBODIES

The Ii antigens are carbohydrates and are present on the interior structures of the complex red cell oligosaccharides (carbohydrate chains) that also carry the ABH and Lewis antigens. The i antigen is associated with un-branched and the I antigen with branched carbohydrate chain structures. The I antigen is very common and is variably expressed on the red cells of different people. Although the Ii antigen strength varies from person to person, the antigen strength of a normal adult remains relatively constant and is inheritable, though a variation in Ii antigenic expression may occur with age and disease presence. The I antigen is not developed at birth (i.e. all cord blood red cells being I negative).

Anti-I antibodies are usually IgM immunoglobulins, being normally cold reacting (<20°C) agglutinins. As such, they normally have limited clinical significance, though potent auto-anti-I cold reacting antibodies have been identified to be the cause of cold Autoimmune Haemolytic Anaemias (AIHA).

Although usually reacting below 20°C they may be detectable at 37°C by sensitive enzyme and occasionally AHG techniques. As such some anti-I antibodies may cause weak 'non-specific' positive reactions with the A, B and O red cells used for ABO grouping. Anti-I can be identified by the fact that it gives a negative / weaker reaction with group O cord red cell samples*. Anti-I antibodies may be associated with anti-H, as anti-HI, produced by group A$_1$ and A$_1$B people who have low levels of H antigen. This acts is a 'combined' antibody, only reacting with red cells that express both H and I antigen specificities. Anti-i antibodies are rarely produced, but have been reported to be present in the serum/plasma of some infectious mononucleosis patients.

* Note: Although cord cells are I antigen negative they are frequently also only weakly H reactive and therefore differentiation of anti-H, anti-HI and anti-I specificities based on the use of cord cells should be viewed with caution.

THE "MINOR" BLOOD GROUP SYSTEMS

The blood group systems outlined above are those recognised to be of the greatest importance, either clinically and/or practically, as most antibodies encountered in hospital Blood Banks will belong to one of these systems. There are however a number of other 'minor' blood group systems which may be important and whose antigen frequency varies between different racial groups. Some of these are represented in the following table:

NAME OF BLOOD GROUP SYSTEM	ANTIBODIES
Diego	Anti-Di^a / Anti-Di^b/ Anti-Wr^a / Anti-Wr^b
Cartwright	Anti-Yt^a / Anti-Yt^b
Dombrock	Anti-Do^a / Anti-Do^b
Colton	Anti-Co^a / Anti-Co^b
Indian	Anti-In^a / Anti-In^b

Antibodies to these blood group antigen specificities pose a variety of practical problems:

1. The antigen frequencies of many of these blood group systems vary greatly between different ethnic backgrounds. Some of the antigens are only of low frequency in certain populations and as a result the production of certain antibody specificities may be virtually restricted to peoples of a specific ethnic group. Information regarding the patient's ethnic background may therefore be an important factor in helping to elucidate some of these antibody specificities.
2. The presence or absence of the antigens of many of these 'minor blood group systems' is not usually shown on the antigen profiles of antibody screening or antibody identification panels as they are not routinely tested for. Therefore, positive results obtained might not fit any of the antigen specificity patterns on the 'antigen profile sheet' and the reactions may appear 'non-specific'.
3. The antibodies to minor blood groups are frequently produced by people who have also produced other antibody specificities and are present in complex antibody mixtures. This makes elucidation of the antibody specificity even more difficult.

As a result of the above practical problems, blood samples suspected of containing antibodies to the 'minor' blood group system antigens should be referred to a reference laboratory.

HIGH AND LOW FREQUENCY ANTIGENS

Some patients may produce antibodies to low frequency ("private") antigens, i.e. those which are found on the red cells of less than 1% of the population and are not part of an established blood group system. Because these antigens are rare, antibodies to low frequency antigens are not usually detected by antibody screening tests as the antigens are not normally present on these red cell samples, but may be detected by chance when crossmatching. Obviously it is not a problem obtaining compatible blood for these cases but the identification of the antibody specificity may be difficult and will need to be referred to a reference laboratory. Additionally, these antibodies may be found when investigating a case of HDFN. The maternal serum/plasma is non-reactive against antibody identification red cell samples, however the serum/plasma gives a positive reaction with the father's red cells. Antibodies to low frequency antigens are commonly described as being 'naturally occurring' and different examples occasionally occur together in the same serum/plasma. There have been a number of low frequency antigens described, e.g. Sw^a, Wu, Pt^a, etc., most of which have been reported to not be clinically important.

High frequency ("public") antigens are defined as those antigens which are found to be present on the red cells of the vast majority of the population (>99%) and do not form part of an established blood group system. A patient who forms an antibody reactive against one of the high frequency antigens is likely to give positive reactions with all red cell samples used for both antibody detection and identification although the DAT / auto-control will be negative, indicating that the reactions are caused by an alloantibody and not by an autoantibody. It is normally very difficult to identify the antibody specificity and find compatible antigen negative blood for these patients and may require blood held only in a 'rare phenotype' frozen blood bank. A large number of high frequency antigens have been described, e.g. Vel, Lan, Jr^a, Ok^a, Sd^a. Some antibodies to high frequency antigens are clinically significant, being capable of causing immediate severe haemolytic transfusion reactions and HDFN.

In practice, the finding of compatible blood for a patient with an antibody active against a high frequency antigen belonging to one of the blood group systems, e.g. Kp^b, Lu^b, may be just as difficult. The ethnic origin of the antibody producer may give an early indication as to the possible specificity of these antibodies, since the absence of a high frequency antigen, although still rare, is more frequently encountered in certain populations. For example, anti-Fy3, anti-U and anti-Js^b are more frequently seen in peoples of African extraction, due to a higher proportion these people having the rare Fy(a-b-), U- and Js(a+b-) phenotypes, whereas anti-Jr^a and anti-In^b antibodies are more frequently seen in people of Asian extraction, due to these people having the rare Jr(a-) and In(a+b-) phenotype.

High titre - low affinity antibodies

Antibodies to one of the high frequency antigens known as Kn^a ('Knops') are of the type referred to as 'high titre - low avidity' or HTLA antibodies. These antibodies cause little or no red cell destruction, but a great deal of frustration in trying to identify them.

Antibodies to the Chido/Rodgers high frequency 'antigens' are actually directed at the complement protein C4, which is found in varying amounts on red cells and therefore these antibodies react weakly with some red cells and not at all with others.

Possible absence of high frequency antigens (rare phenotype presence) that are associated with people of different ethnic backgrounds

ETHNIC ORIGIN OF PATIENT WITH ANTIBODY	INCREASED POSSIBILITY OF	
	RED CELL PHENOTYPE	ANTIBODY SPECIFICITY
African	Fy(a-b-)	Anti-Fy3
	U- (S-s-)	Anti-U
	Kp(a+b-)	Anti-Kp^b
	Js(a+b-)	Anti-Js^b
Asian	Jr(a-)	Anti-Jr^a
	In(a+b-)	Anti-In^b
Caucasian	K+k-	Anti-k
	Vel-	Anti-Vel
	Yt(a-b+)	Anti-Yt^a
	Kp(a+b-)	Anti-Kp^b

The following tables of the more common antibody specificities and how they react summarises the important features. It is occasionally useful to have copies of these tables, or something similar, to refer to when performing antibody identification tests.

SUMMARY OF THE ANTIBODY REACTIONS OF THE MAJOR BLOOD GROUP SYSTEMS

SYSTEM	ANTIBODY	ORIGIN *	Ig CLASS	ANTIBODY REACTIVITY:			
				Sal 20°C	Sal 37°C	AHG 37°C	Enz 37°C
ABO	Anti-A	NO / I	IgM	Yes	Yes	Yes	Yes
	Anti-B	NO / I	IgM	Yes	Yes	Yes	Yes
	Anti-A,B	NO / I	IgM(G)	Yes	Yes	Yes	Yes
	Anti-A$_1$	NO / I	IgM(G)	Yes	Rare	Rare	Rare
Rh	Anti-D	I	IgG(M)	Rare	Some	Yes	Yes
	Anti-C	I	IgG(M)	Rare	Some	Yes	Yes
	Anti-c	I	IgG	Rare	Rare	Yes	Yes
	Anti-E	NO / I	IgG(M)	Some	Some	Yes	Yes
	Anti-e	I	IgG	Rare	Rare	Yes	Yes
MNS	Anti-M	NO / (I)	IgM	Yes	Rare	Some	No
	Anti-N	NO / (I)	IgM	Yes	Rare	Rare	No
	Anti-S	I	IgG	Rare	Rare	Yes	No
	Anti-s	I	IgG	Rare	Rare	Yes	No
P	Anti-P$_1$	NO / (I)	IgM	Yes	Rare	Rare	Some
Kell	Anti-K	I	IgG	Rare	Some	Yes	Some
	Anti-k	I	IgG	Rare	Rare	Yes	Some
Duffy	Anti-Fy^a	I	IgG	Rare	Rare	Yes	No
	Anti-Fy^b	I	IgG	Rare	Rare	Yes	No
Kidd	Anti-Jk^a	I	IgG	Rare	Rare	Yes	Some
	Anti-Jk^b	I	IgG	Rare	Rare	Yes	Some
Lewis	Anti-Le^a	NO / (I)	IgM(G)	Yes	Yes	Yes	Yes
	Anti-Le^b	NO / (I)	IgM(G)	Yes	Yes	Yes	Yes
Lutheran	Anti-Lu^a	NO / (I)	IgM(G)	Yes	Rare	Some	Some
	Anti-Lu^b	NO / (I)	IgG/IgM	Rare	Rare	Yes	Some

Origin *:
NO = 'Naturally Occurring' antibody, i.e. stimulated in the absence of transfusion or pregnancy.
I = Immune, i.e. stimulated as a result of pregnancy or transfusion immunisation.

DETAILS OF SOME ANTIBODY SPECIFICITIES ENCOUNTERED IN BLOOD GROUP SEROLOGY

ANTIBODY SPECIFICITY	REACTS BEST BY	ANTIGEN FREQUENCY *	CLINICAL SIGNIFICANCE	
			HDFN	TR
D	Enzyme, AHG	85%	+	+
C	Enzyme, AHG	70%	Rare	Rare
c	Enzyme, AHG	80%	+	+
E	Enzyme, AHG	28%	+	+
e	Enzyme, AHG	98%	+	+
C^w	Enzyme, AHG	3%	+	x
Le^a	Enzyme, AHG, Saline	22%	x	+
Le^b	Enzyme, AHG, Saline	72%	x	?
Le^{a+b}	Enzyme, AHG, Saline	94%	x	+
P_1	Saline	79%	x	?
I	Saline	100%	x	Rare
M	Saline (LISS)	78%	Rare	(+)
N	Saline (LISS)	72%	Rare	Rare
S	AHG, Saline	55%	Rare	+
s	AHG	89%	Rare	+
U	AHG	99.9%	+	+
Wr^a	AHG	<1%	+	+
Fy^a	AHG	66%	+	+
Fy^b	AHG	83%	NR	+
Jk^a	AHG	77%	+	+
Jk^b	AHG	72%	+	+
K	AHG	9%	+	+
k	AHG	99.8%	+	+
Lu^a	Saline, AHG	8%	NR	X
Lu^b	AHG	99.8%	(+)	+

Key:
* UK Whites
HDFN = Haemolytic Disease of the Fetus/Newborn
TR = Transfusion Reaction
+ = Occurs
x = Does not occur
? = Sometimes
(+) = Mild
NR = Not reported.

SUMMARY DETAILS FOR SOME OF THE BLOOD GROUP SYSTEMS

NAME	SYSTEM SYMBOL	SYSTEM NUMBER	ISBT SYMBOL	NUMBER OF ANTIGENS	MAJOR ANTIGENS	CHROMOSOME LOCATION	MEMBRANE STRUCTURE
ABO	ABO	001	ABO	4	A, A_1, B	9 (q34.1-q34.2)	Carbohydrate
MNS	MN	002	MNS	38	M, N, S, s	4 (q28-q31)	GPA GPB
P	P	003	P1	1	P_1	22 (q11.2-qter)	Glycolipid
Rh	Rh	004	RH	45	D, C, c, E, e	1 (p36.2-p34)	Proteins
Lutheran	Lu	005	LU	18	Lu^a, Lu^b	19 (q12-q13)	Ig superfamily (IgSF)
Kell	K	006	KEL	21	K, k, Kp^a, Kp^b, Js^a, Js^b	7 (q33)	Glycoprotein
Lewis	Le	007	LE	3	Le^a, Le^b	19 (p13.3)	Carbohydrate
Duffy	Fy	008	FY	6	Fy^a, Fy^b	1 (q22-q23)	RBC chemokine receptor
Kidd	Jk	009	JK	3	Jk^a, Jk^b	18 (q11-q12)	Urea transporter
Diego	Di	010	DI	4	Di^a, Di^b, Wr^a, Wr^b	17 (q12-q21)	Glycoprotein (Band 3)
Yt (Cartwright)	Yt	011	YT	2	Yt^a, Yt^b	7 (q22)	Acetylcholinesterase (AChE)
Xg	Xg	012	XG	1	Xg^a	X (p22.32)	Glycoprotein
Scianna	Sc	013	SC	3	Sc1, Sc2	1 (p36.2-p22.1)	Glycoprotein
Dombrock	Do	014	DO	5	Do^a, Do^b	12 (p13.3-p13.2)	GP1 - linked protein
Colton	Co	015	CO	3	Co^a, Co^b	7 (p14)	Aquaporin -1 (AQP-CHIP)
Landsteiner-Wiener	LW	016	LW	3	LW^a, LW^b	19 (p13.2-cent)	Ig superfamily (IgSF)
Chido / Rodgers	Ch/Rg	017	CH/RG	9	Ch, Rg	6 (p21.3)	C4A C4B
Hh	H	018	H	1	H	19 (q13.3)	Carbohydrate
Kx	Kx	019	XK	1	Kx	X (p21.1)	Glycoprotein
Gerbich	Ge	020	GE	7	Ge2, Ge3	2 (q14-q21)	Glycophorin C Glycophorin D
Cromer	Cromer	021	CROM	10	Cr^a, Tc^a	1 (q32)	Decay accelerating factor (DAF)
Knops	Kn	022	KN	5	Kn^a, Kn^b, Yk^a	1 (q32)	Glycoprotein CR1 (CD35)
Indian	In	023	IN	2	In^a, In^b	11 (p13)	Glycoprotein CD44
OK	Ok	024	OK	1	Ok^a	19 (p13.3)	Ig superfamily (CD147)
RAPH	RAPH	025	RAPH	1	MER2	11 (p15.5)	-
John Milton Hagen	JMH	026	JMH	1	JMH	15 (q22.3-q23)	CDw108

QUESTIONS - SECTION 10

1. List the 'major blood group systems' and their principal antigens.

2. List the antigens that are destroyed by proteolytic enzymes, such as papain.

3. Why is anti-k such a rare antibody?

4. Why is anti-K such a common antibody?

5. What blood group donations should be selected for a group A Rh D positive patient with anti-Fy^a reactive by AHG at 37°C and anti-A_1 reactive by saline techniques at 20°C?

6. How does an antibody to a high frequency antigen normally react in pre-transfusion tests? How is its specificity identified?

7. Which of the major blood group system antibodies are not normally clinically significant?

8. Which is the most common Duffy genotype in White and Black populations?

9. Which of the following antibodies are classified as 'clinically significant'?

    a. Anti-Jk^a
    b. Anti-Fy^b
    c. Anti-M (reactive at 37°C)
    d. Anti-Lu^b

10. Why is it possible for a RBC Lewis group to change from Le(a-b+) to Le(a-b-)?

SECTION 11

HAEMOLYTIC DISEASE OF THE FETUS/NEWBORN

The condition now known as Haemolytic Disease of the Fetus/Newborn (HDFN) was shown to be caused by maternal antibody destroying the fetal red cells by Levine and Stetson and reported in an American journal in 1939 under the title 'an unusual case of intragroup incompatibility.'

The first reported cases of HDFN were all caused by anti-D and this antibody is the most frequent cause of severe HDFN despite the continuing routine use of anti-D immunoglobulin therapy.

AETIOLOGY OF HDFN

HDFN occurs when maternal IgG antibodies cross the placenta and bind to the corresponding antigen on the fetal red cells.

A positive direct antiglobulin test (DAT) with the red cells of a newborn infant does not on its own establish the diagnosis of HDFN, since a positive DAT may not necessarily result in a decreased fetal red cell survival. Evidence of increased red cell destruction is also required but in practice, clinical evidence of decreased red cell survival in a newborn infant is very difficult to establish. This is due to the fact that virtually every newborn infant shows a rise in bilirubin levels during the first 2-3 days of life, as well as a progressive fall in haemoglobin during the first few weeks of life. Clinical signs of HDFN include:

- Jaundice (though this may have a non-immunological cause).
- Anaemia (excessive fall in haemoglobin level).
- Enlargement of the liver and spleen.

The severity of the disease ranges from mild anaemia to stillbirth. This depends essentially on the number of fetal red cells destroyed by the maternal antibody, and the ability of the fetus to compensate by an increased production of new red cells, which is related to the age of the fetus.

HDFN may therefore result if both of the following occur at the same time:

- The mother has a 37°C active IgG red cell alloantibody (sub-class IgG1 and/or IgG3). IgM antibodies do not cross the placenta, therefore only IgG antibodies are capable of causing HDFN. The presence of a 37°C IgG reactive antibody in the mother is rare, since it requires prior sensitisation.
- The corresponding antigen is present on the fetal red cells (the gene for which is paternally derived). The presence of the antigen on the fetal red cells must by definition indicate that the fetus is heterozygous, having received the gene to produce the antigen from the father, but the mother must be antigen negative since she has produced the antibody. The father may be either homozygous, in which case all of his future offspring are likely to be affected by the maternal antibody, or heterozygous, in which case potentially 50% of his future children will be affected by the maternal antibody.

ORIGINS OF THE MATERNAL ANTIBODY

To be capable of causing HDFN, either a previous transfusion and/or pregnancy must have stimulated the woman to have produced an IgG 37°C reactive immune antibody.

Stimulation by a previous transfusion

This is the most common cause of HDFN occurring in the first pregnancy (i.e. the woman having been transfused prior to her pregnancy) and is associated with HDFN due to non-RhD specificity antibodies, as all D negative female patients in the UK should only receive D negative and where possible K negative blood (see below). In addition, transfusion is an effective method of stimulating the production of some non-Rh specificity antibodies, i.e. Duffy and Kidd. The production of any antibody following a transfusion will of course only be significant in causing HDFN if the woman subsequently has a baby that inherits the corresponding gene from the father, resulting in the fetal red cells being antigen positive.

Stimulation by previous pregnancy

Maternal antibody is stimulated by transplacental feto-maternal haemorrhage (FMH). The fetal red cells, which are capable of surviving a normal life span in the maternal circulation, carry paternally derived antigens that are foreign to the mother and are therefore capable of immunising her to produce an immune antibody response. Small numbers of fetal red cells cross the placenta throughout pregnancy, however the number of fetal red cells detectable in the maternal circulation is greater towards the end of the pregnancy. A traumatic delivery, i.e. manual placental removal and Caesarean Section, results in a greater chance of fetal cells being transferred into the maternal circulation. Stillbirth and abortion can also result in trans-placental haemorrhage. Since fetal red cells enter the maternal circulation towards the end of the pregnancy / immediately after delivery, any stimulated IgG antibody produced normally only affects the second or subsequent pregnancies. However, due to the fact that the antibody specificity is essentially paternally stimulated, assuming that the woman has further children to the same man, there is a strong likelihood that the antibody will affect at least some, or all, of these children. The majority of antibodies stimulated by pregnancy are Rh specificities, especially anti-D, anti-C+D and anti-c. This is due to the strong immunogenicity of the Rh antigens (especially D) and the fact that approximately 1 in 10 pregnancies in Whites involve a D negative mother with a D positive fetus. Stimulation of an antibody via pregnancy is more likely to result in HDFN as:

1. The antibody specificity is usually within Rh, e.g. anti-D and anti-C+D.
2. The antibody is stimulated by paternally derived antigens and as such is more likely to be related to causing HDFN in subsequent pregnancies.

POSSIBLE PROTECTION BY ABO INCOMPATIBILITY

The potential for antibody stimulation appears to be related to the life span (and clearance) of the fetal red cells in the maternal circulation. Therefore maternal ABO blood group antibodies may provide some 'protection' by removing ABO incompatible fetal red cells from the maternal circulation. For example, if the mother is group O and the fetus is group A (i.e. genetic *AO*), then the maternal anti-A,B will react with the fetal red cells destroying or removing them from the maternal circulation. This mechanism will obviously vary in its effectiveness dependant upon a number of factors including the amount and frequency of fetal bleeds, fetal antigen development and the maternal antibody.

TRANSFER OF ANTIBODY FROM MOTHER TO FETUS

In humans, the transfer of antibody from mother to fetus takes place only via the placenta. The only blood group reactive immunoglobulin capable of placental transfer is IgG (mainly IgG1 and IgG3), due to a placental transfer factor which is located on the Fc portion of the molecule (see Section 1: Antigen - Antibody Reactions).

At delivery, the concentration of IgG tends to be higher in the infant's serum/plasma than in the mother's serum/plasma. This difference is due to the fact that IgG is transferred more readily from the mother to the fetus than from the fetus to the mother. Maternal antibody remains in the circulation of the infant with a half-life of approximately 23 days.

ANTIBODY SPECIFICITIES THAT CAUSE HDFN

ABO
Although the anti-A of a group B and the anti-B of a group A individual is normally predominantly IgM, the serum/plasma of many group O women may contain a high titre IgG anti-A,B. Therefore, group A and group B children of group O mothers (which account for approximately 15% of all pregnancies) are theoretically at risk from HDFN due to the maternal IgG antibody. As a result, ABO incompatibility between mother and fetus is common, (mother O, baby A) and can give rise to jaundice of the newborn and sometimes a positive DAT. However, true ABO HDFN due to maternal IgG anti-A or anti-B, requiring more than phototherapy treatment, is rare in the UK. Mild jaundice due to ABO incompatibility occurs in only approximately 1 in 150 births (or approximately 0.67% of newborn infants) and of these, very few infants (approximately 1 in 3,000) require any treatment. This effect is due to the fact that fetal A and B antigens are not fully developed at birth as well as the presence of non-red cell and secreted A or B substances in the fetus and placenta, which is capable of neutralising the maternal antibody. The DAT of the infant's red cells is therefore frequently negative or only weakly positive in cases of ABO HDFN and the estimation of the presence and titre of maternal IgG anti-A,B as a prediction of the severity of ABO HDFN is of little value.

Rh
The major cause of severe HDFN is anti-D, despite the use of 'immunoprophylaxis' for the past 30 years; however the number of cases is now quite small and death from Rh HDFN in the UK is currently quoted as being in the order of 1 in 20,000 pregnancies. Apart from anti-D the other Rh antibody likely to cause severe HDFN is anti-c. Rh antibodies such as anti-E, anti-Ce, anti-e and anti-C^w have been reported to have caused HDFN but usually are less severe, often not requiring any treatment other than phototherapy.

In Rh mediated cases, if sufficient antibody molecules are bound to the red cells they will be destroyed by the fetal reticuloendothelial system, which might lead to anaemia. If severe this could cause death, through heart failure, as the heart has to work harder to pump the decreased numbers of red cells around the fetal circulation.

Other antibody specificities
In general, as well as anti-D and anti-c, anti-K has the greatest potential to cause HDFN, though anti-Fy^a, anti-Jk^a and anti-C^w have also been identified to cause clinically significant HDFN. The antibody specificities anti-M, anti-N, anti-S, anti-s and anti-Lu^b are reported to rarely cause HDFN. In addition, other rarer IgG 37°C reactive antibody

specificities may have the capability of causing HDFN, though their potential clinical importance needs to be assessed on an individual basis.

Anti-Le^a, anti-Le^b, anti-P$_1$, anti-I and high titre-low avidity (HTLA) antibodies have not been implicated in causing HDFN. Anti-Lu^a and anti-Fy^b have not been reported to cause HDFN.

Most examples of anti-K found in pregnancy are the result of transfusion not a feto-maternal haemorrhage. Because of this it is now recommended that women of child-bearing potential (under 60 years of age) are transfused with K negative red cells wherever possible, to reduce the number of women sensitised and thereby HDFN caused by anti-K. Anti-K can be the cause HDFN but unlike Rh antibodies, anti-K binds to red cell precursors in the bone marrow and seems to suppress red cell production that leads to anaemia. As there is little or no actual red cell destruction bilirubin levels are not raised and treatment is for anaemia only.

If the fetus survives there may be problems after birth; initially because of anaemia but then there is a risk of neurological damage due to high bilirubin levels. Whilst *in utero* the bilirubin from destroyed red cells is removed by the mother's liver, but once born the infant is unable to cope with the bilirubin (because of the lack of the liver enzyme that conjugates it) and therefore the levels of bilirubin in the blood increase. Although bilirubin binds to albumin, once this is saturated it will bind to lipids in the brain, which can then lead to brain damage (kernicterus). Therefore treatment of HDFN might involve one or a combination of the following:

- Intrauterine transfusion (IUT), to prevent the fetus becoming too anaemic
- Immediate exchange transfusion after delivery, to treat anaemia
- Exchange transfusion to prevent the bilirubin becoming too high (by removing the plasma containing the bilirubin, as well as the sensitised red cells that are 'potential' bilirubin)
- Possible simple 'top-up' transfusions several days post delivery to correct anaemia
- In mild cases ultraviolet light (photo) therapy

LABORATORY TESTING FOR THE PREVENTION OF HDFN

Published guidelines recommend that all women should be tested twice during their pregnancy, at first booking (normally 12-16 weeks) and, if no red cell alloantibody specificity is detected, again at approximately 28-30 weeks. This test system recognises that all women, not just those who are D negative, carry a significant chance of producing an antibody capable of causing HDFN (e.g. anti-c, anti-K). These specificities may otherwise be missed if women are only tested once during early pregnancy. The objectives of the serological testing of the blood samples from pregnant women are to:

- Identify pregnancies at risk of fetal and neonatal HDFN.
- Identify D- women who may need anti-D immunoglobulin prophylaxis.
- Provide antigen negative blood swiftly for obstetric emergencies.

At the time of booking (12-16 weeks) a sample for ABO, RhD typing and antibody screening should be collected from every woman. Tests for HIV, hepatitis B, syphilis and rubella antibodies should also be offered at this time. If no red cell antibodies are present then a further sample should be tested at 28-30 weeks, for ABO, RhD and an antibody screen. All techniques used should be well established and validated by good laboratory methods, according to published guidelines.

If the antibody screen is positive the antibody should be identified. Women who have anti-D, -c or anti-K should be re-tested every 4 weeks during the first 2 trimesters of pregnancy and from 28 weeks every 2 weeks. Those with other antibodies (e.g. anti-Fy^a) are tested again at 28 weeks and further testing is dependent on these results. If the specificity is either anti-D (-C+D, -D+E, -C+D+E) or anti-c the level of antibody can be determined by 'automated antibody quantification' (see below). Anti-K and/or other specificities that are known to be capable of causing HDFN are titrated by IAT to determine the 'antibody titre'.

Possibility of HDFN due to the presence of maternal anti-D:
- below 4 IU/mL : HDFN is unlikely to occur
- levels of 4-15 IU/mL are associated with mild to moderate risk of disease
- levels above 15 IU/mL are associated with a high risk of HDFN

Note: An increase in anti-D level of 50% or greater over the previous result indicates a significant rate of increase in the amount of antibody, irrespective of the stage in the gestation. Published data has indicated that this is especially important when the anti-D level increases to over 10 IU/mL. For values of <0.l IU/mL it is important to check to identify if prophylactic anti-D immunoglobulin has been given to the woman.

Possibility of HDFN due to the presence of maternal anti-c:
- below 7.5 IU/mL : little risk of HDFN occurring
- levels of 7.5-20 IU/mL are associated with a moderate risk of disease
- levels above 20 IU/mL are associated with a high risk of HDFN.

Titrations of anti-K are performed regularly, unless it can be shown that the 'father' is K negative and then follow-up tests are carried out only at 28 weeks. Estimation of the amount of antibody provides an indication of the possible severity of the effects of the maternal antibody on the fetus, since the greater the amount of antibody present in the maternal serum/plasma the more likely it is to cross the placenta and possibly affect the fetus. There is some correlation between the titre and the severity of HDFN and titres greater than 32 are considered significant. However, anti-K may result in severe HDFN regardless of the maternal titre score and as such, if the partner and/or fetus is identified to be K+, referral to a specialist fetal unit may be advised. Other antibodies, such as anti-Fy^a, can cause mild or sometimes moderate disease. Titrations should be performed and values less than 32 are unlikely to result in significant disease; levels greater than 32 are considered significant.

Quantification of maternal antibody concentration

The detection of anti-D or anti-c in the maternal serum/plasma requires that the antibody is quantified by an automated technique. The method is reproducible and the results correlate reasonably well with the likelihood of HDFN. This technique is only reliable however for anti-D (as well as anti-D+C and anti-D+C+E specificities) and anti-c antibodies. The technique involves automatic serum/plasma dilution, the use of a reaction enhancing agent (bromelin) and a red cell aggregating agent (methyl cellulose) to increase the reaction speed. A standardised end-point reading is obtained by means of a spectrophotometer. By the use of a British standard, the results can be reported in International Units (IU) per mL (5 IU/mL of anti-D is equivalent to 1µg of anti-D protein as estimated by RIA).

Diagrammatic representation of the basic general layout for a (single-channel) analyser for antibody quantification

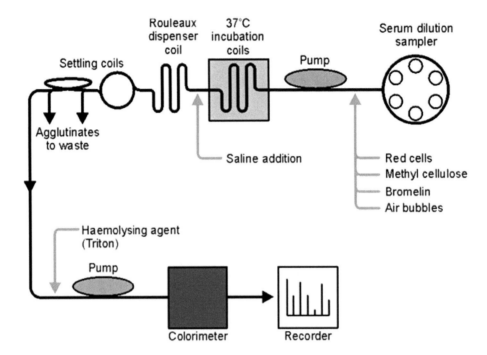

One of the major roles of Rh antibody quantification during pregnancy, especially since there is a relatively poor correlation with outcome in the majority of cases which fall into the mid-range values, is as an indicator to the obstetrician and paediatrician as to the clinical management of the pregnancy. If there is a significant amount of antibody in the serum/plasma of a woman, referral to a specialist fetal monitoring unit is recommended, enabling a more informed decision as to the potential effects on the fetus to be made, i.e. typically by the use of Ultrasonography or Doppler velocity.

Tests performed at and after delivery

At delivery of an infant of any mother with atypical antibodies a cord blood sample should be collected for an Hb and DAT. If the Hb is low, an immediate exchange transfusion might be needed. If the initial Hb is normal and the DAT is positive the bilirubin should be monitored and if it becomes elevated an exchange might then be necessary.

If IUTs have been performed because the mother has a very high level of anti-D then D negative blood would have been transfused. Cord blood samples might then type as D negative as the infants own (D positive) red cells have been replaced with the D negative donor blood. However it is important that the Hb and bilirubin levels are still closely monitored as the infant could well become anaemic or jaundiced as their own D positive cells are still being produced.

PREVENTION OF HDFN USING ANTI-D IMMUNOGLOBULIN

If an injection of anti-D immunoglobulin is given to a woman who is D negative, but who has not been stimulated to produce anti-D, at the time she might be exposed to fetal D positive red cells crossing over the placenta, those 'foreign' cells will be removed from her circulation before they can stimulate her immune system to produce anti-D. Feto-maternal haemorrhage (FMH), most commonly occurs at delivery but can also happen during pregnancy due to abdominal injury, external version of the fetus etc. They can also occur in ectopic pregnancies, intrauterine deaths, threatened, spontaneous or therapeutic abortions. Anti-D Ig should therefore be given to all RhD negative women within 72 hours of any of these events. Before 20 weeks gestation a 250 IU dose is given, after 20 weeks a minimum of 500 IU, which will clear up to 4ml of fetal blood, is given. A blood sample should be taken however to see if there has been a large FMH and extra anti-D Ig is needed; a Kleihauer acid elution test is usually used. If the haemorrhage is judged to be greater than 4ml, then the size of the bleed should be estimated to determine the dose of anti-D required. Guidelines recommend that a flow cytometry method should be used to quantify bleeds larger than 2ml as this method is more accurate than the Kleihauer technique.

The Kleihauer acid elution method requires the examination of a blood film made from the maternal sample. The film is treated with a low pH, acid, buffer to elute the adult haemoglobin from the maternal cells leaving the fetal cells stained by the eosin counter stain. The film is then examined microscopically and if less than 4 fetal cells are seen per standard low-power field, it is assumed the FMH is less than 4ml. However if fetal cells are seen in every low power field then the ratio of maternal to fetal cells is estimated and the size of the FMH, in ml of fetal red cells, is calculated using the formula:

$$\frac{2400}{\text{Ratio of adult : fetal cells}}$$

Flow cytometry also provides an accurate and reproducible means of quantifying D+ fetal red cells in a maternal D negative blood sample. The method is used to confirm results obtained by the Kleihauer method, especially those indicating a large fetal bleed. Both direct and indirect methods can be employed. The direct method uses a monoclonal anti-D reagent conjugated with fluorochrome whereas the indirect method involves treating the maternal sample with an IgG anti-D (which binds to the fetal D+ red cells) and then the sample is treated with an anti-IgG antibody labelled with a fluorescent dye.

Despite many years of use of anti-D Ig there are still about 1.5% of at risk mothers producing anti-D, mainly during the last trimester of pregnancy rather than at delivery. To reduce this incidence the National Institute for Clinical Excellence (NICE) has recommended the use of 'routine antenatal prophylaxis' using anti-D immunoglobulin. Anti-D immunoglobulin injections are given during the third trimester, either as two injections at 28 and 34 weeks, or as a single (larger dose) injection at 28 weeks, to all D negative women to prevent them forming anti-D late in pregnancy. Anti-D Ig should still be given in the normal way following the delivery of an Rh D positive infant.

From a laboratory view point this can present a problem as the injected anti-D can be detected in serological tests, weakly reactive by IAT. If antibody screening is required post anti-D injection 'rr (cde/cde) screening cells' can be used instead of the usual D positive screening cells, to detect the presence of other antibodies. Also infants born to mothers who have received anti-D immunoglobulin might have a weak direct antiglobulin test but have no signs of any increased red cell destruction. It has been reported that this might be found in up to 8% of infants born to D negative mothers having had anti-D injections. With the widespread of anti-D immunoglobulin therapy HDFN may become even more of a rarity than now.

Potential feto-maternal sensitising episodes occurring during pregnancy following which Rh D negative women should receive anti-D Ig:
- Therapeutic termination of pregnancy
- Ectopic pregnancy
- Spontaneous (complete or incomplete) abortion (>12 weeks)
- Amniocentesis
- Chorionic villus sampling
- Fetal blood sampling
- Intrauterine bleeding (>12 weeks) / antepartum haemorrhage
- External cephalic version of the fetus
- Closed abdominal surgery
- Intrauterine death
- Miscarriage / stillbirth
- Manual removal of placenta
- Abdominal trauma

A 'natural' red cell bleed from the fetus to the mother is not necessarily associated with obvious symptoms (e.g. such as pain and/or bleeding). Such 'silent' bleeds are not uncommon and occur more frequently in the third trimester. All invasive procedures are associated with risks to the fetus as well as causing possible feto-maternal bleeding, which could stimulate antibody production and may also cause a rise in the titre of an existing antibody, thereby aggravating the problem.

See also the 'Guidelines for blood grouping and red cell antibody testing during pregnancy' and Handbook of Transfusion Medicine, 4th Edition p53 (see: Sources of Additional Information for reference details).

Intrauterine transfusion (IUT)
This is a rare treatment option, however when the fetus is severely affected in early pregnancy, intrauterine transfusion may be the only available treatment. The red cell infusion can be given either via intravascular, into the umbilical vein, the process being directed by ultrasonography or via an intraperitoneal transfusion where the red cells are injected into the peritoneal cavity from where they are taken up by the fetal blood stream. The blood selected should be antigen negative for the maternal antibody specificity and crossmatch negative at 37°C by IAT using the mother's serum/plasma and irradiated before use to avoid the risk of graft versus host disease.

Intrauterine transfusion is also used for the treatment of Neonatal Alloimmune Thrombocytopenia (NAITP). NAITP occurs due to the presence of an IgG anti-platelet antibody in the maternal circulation, with the respective antigen being present on fetal platelets (paternally derived). Over 95% of NAITP cases are due to the platelet antibody specificity anti-HPA-1a or 5b. This condition carries a high risk of intracranial haemorrhage (50% of which can occur before birth). Hyperconcentrates containing 2-4,000x10^9/L of (antigen negative) platelets per pack are transfused.

Exchange transfusion
The technique, performed shortly after delivery, involves withdrawing blood from the infant using a syringe and re-injecting fresh red cells intermittently, by means of a three-way connection to a plastic catheter passed into the umbilical vein. The blood selected should be antigen negative for the maternal antibody specificity and crossmatch

negative at 37°C by IAT using the mother's serum/plasma (and irradiated if the baby has received a previous intrauterine transfusion). Exchange transfusion has two main differences over a simple ('top-up') transfusion:

- It removes some of the antibody coated fetal red cells before they are destroyed, replacing them with red cells that survive normally.
- It removes some of the bilirubin, reducing the risk of kernicterus and possible brain damage due to the effects of high concentrations of unconjugated bilirubin.

For further information on red cell products provided for intrauterine and exchange transfusion procedures see Section 14: Blood and Blood Products - Selection of products for neonatal use, and Components for use in intrauterine / exchange transfusions of neonates and infants under one year.

QUESTIONS - SECTION 11

1. What antibody specificity causes the most serious / major HDFN? Why is this?

2. Which blood group system is the most frequent cause of HDFN? Why is this?

3. What levels of anti-D is associated with:
   - Low risk of HDFN?
   - Mild to moderate risk of HDFN?
   - High risk of HDFN?

4. When should anti-D immunoglobulin be given?

5. What test is performed to identify the amount of a feto-maternal bleed?

6. Feto-maternal haemorrhage most commonly occurs at delivery. What other conditions can lead to a feto-maternal haemorrhage?

7. Should anti-D prophylaxis be offered to an Rh D negative mother with anti-D who has delivered an Rh D positive baby? Explain the reasons for your answer?

8. Following the detection of a 37°C IAT reactive antibody in an antenatal blood sample, what further action should be taken?

9. What options are available to treat severe HDFN?

10. How does anti-K cause HDFN?

IMMUNE HAEMOLYTIC ANAEMIAS

THE DIRECT ANTIGLOBULIN TEST

The DAT is used in the investigation of cases of suspected immune red cell destruction. However a positive DAT, in itself, is not diagnostic of a *haemolytic anaemia*, as there also has to be evidence of increased red cell destruction, such as a low Hb, raised reticulocyte count, reduced haptoglobins, raised bilirubin, raised LDH. A DAT should be performed using a polyspecific AHG reagent that contains both anti-IgG and anti-C3, as these are often found on red cells from patients with immune red cell destruction. When investigating a case of suspected autoimmune haemolytic anaemia monospecific reagents anti-IgG, anti-C3d, anti-IgM and anti-IgA should be included.

AUTOIMMUNE HAEMOLYTIC ANAEMIAS

As already stated, red cell antibodies produced as a result of transfusion and/or pregnancy can cause either the destruction of red cells if incompatible blood is transfused, a Haemolytic Transfusion Reaction (HTR), or the destruction of fetal red cells, Haemolytic Disease of the Fetus/Newborn (HDFN). However, some patients produce autoantibodies, directed against their own red cells, which can lead to an increased rate of cell destruction – an Autoimmune Haemolytic Anaemia (AIHA).

AIHA is a relatively rare condition usually found secondary to other clinical disorders especially haematological malignancies. Patients with AIHA may present on admission with a very low Hb, sometimes <5 g/dL, and require an immediate transfusion to maintain their Hb until other treatment has time to suppress the increased rate of red cell destruction. Autoimmune Haemolytic Anaemias can be divided into 4 categories:
- Warm AIHA
- Cold AIHA
- Paroxysmal Cold Haemoglobinuria (PCH)
- Drug induced / associated

WARM TYPE AIHA

This is the most common type and is caused by an IgG autoantibody; sometimes the C3 component of complement is also present on the patient's red cells. Therefore the DAT is positive with anti-IgG and possibly anti-C3 as well. If the red cells are coated with IgG, destruction takes place in the spleen, but if complement has been activated there might be some more rapid cell destruction in the liver. A diagnosis of 'haemolytic anaemia' can only be made if there is evidence of red cell destruction such as a falling Hb, raised reticulocytes and/or raised bilirubin.

In some cases IgM or IgA antibodies may be found in addition to IgG and very rarely IgA might be present on its own. It is only by using a monospecific anti-IgA AHG reagent that these cases are recognised.

The autoantibodies found in warm AIHA sometimes have a recognisable Rh-related specificity with auto-anti-e or 'e-like' being the most commonly encountered, although a variety of other antibody specificities have also been reported. Grouping cells with a positive DAT due to IgG can be performed using IgM blood typing sera, but those that require an IAT cannot be used as the cells would react with the AHG regardless of their antigen status.

Although some cases of warm AIHA are 'idiopathic', occurring without any obvious underlying cause, most cases of positive DATs now seen are related to haematological malignancies. In a series of cases referred to the NBS Colindale RCI reference laboratory only 5% were idiopathic AIHA, 16% were associated with cases of malignancy and 10% with MDS.

DAT negative AIHA
There have been cases reported where a patient has clinical AIHA but the DAT has been negative. On further investigation some of these have been shown to have IgA on the cell surface but in others it is assumed that either low-affinity autoantibodies are involved or there are low levels of IgG1 or IgG3, that are not detectable in the standard DAT.

Therapeutic immunoglobulins
The use of the therapeutic immunoglobulin preparations, anti-lymphocyte and anti-thymocyte globulins, has resulted in positive DATs as the immunoglobulins 'stick' to the red cells in a non-specific manner.

Positive DAT without cell destruction
A number of patients and donors have a positive DAT with no evidence of increased cell destruction. Reported figures vary from 1 in 3,000 to 1 in 15,000 donors. The reason for the lack of clinical significance might be that the cells are coated with IgG4 molecules that seem not to initiate cell destruction. Some patients with raised IgG levels can also have a weak positive DAT, presumably due to non-specific uptake of their IgG onto their own red cells.

Positive DAT in malaria
The DAT has been reported positive (IgG and/or C3) in some patients with *Plasmodium falciparum* malaria. As haemolysis in malaria is multifactorial it is not clear to what extent it is exacerbated when the DAT is positive.

COLD TYPE AIHA

The antibodies associated with cold AIHA are not usually detected on the cells by the DAT, but C3 is present indicating that an antigen-antibody reaction has taken place. These cases are caused by a cold-reacting IgM autoantibody, often anti-I or anti-i. These antibodies react with the patient's own cells in the peripheral capillaries, such as the finger tips, where the blood might be at 30°C, rather than 37°C. At these lower temperatures the antibody binds to the antigen and initiates the complement cascade. As the blood returns to the warmer parts of the body the antibody elutes from the cells but as the complement cascade has been started it might, in extreme cases, go to completion resulting in intravascular lysis or rapid lysis in the liver. When this happens the patient can present with haemoglobinuria after exposure to the cold. In less extreme cases the complement cascade is halted at the C3 stage and C3d is found on the red cells, which probably have a near normal half-life.

Paroxysmal Cold Haemoglobinuria (PCH)

PCH is usually categorised as a cold type AIHA but is unlike AIHA caused by IgM antibodies. The causative antibody in PCH is bi-phasic, IgG, usually with anti-P specificity; the so-called Donath-Landsteiner antibody. The antibody reacts in the cold and activates complement in the warm leading to haemolysis and haemoglobinuria. The Donath-Landsteiner test is used to detect these antibodies. In this test, group O cells and the serum under investigation are first incubated at $0^{\circ}C$ then at $37^{\circ}C$, with a control incubated only at $37^{\circ}C$. In a positive test, lysis is seen in the tube incubated at both temperatures but not in the one incubated only at $37^{\circ}C$.

Although classically associated with syphilis this condition is now almost always seen in children, often associated with a viral infection. Although it is self-limiting, that is it resolves after a few days, some patients do present with acute haemolysis that requires transfusion. Although P positive blood is tolerated by some patients for others it is necessary to transfuse rare P negative units if the P+ cells are quickly destroyed.

DRUG INDUCED OR DRUG-ASSOCIATED AIHA

A number of drugs (over 100), have been reported to be capable of binding to red cells and initiating an immune response. Although these are frequently reported in the USA, very few cases are reported in the UK. The stimulated antibodies can react with the drug itself or to drug plus membrane components or mainly to the cell membrane. Four mechanisms have been described:

- Drug-dependent antibodies which react mainly against the drug.
  The DAT in these cases is usually positive with IgG and sometimes also with C3. The antibodies only react with drug-coated cells. The drugs involved are mainly the penicillins and cephalosporins. Haemolysis develops slowly but can be life threatening.
- Immune complex mechanism.
  This involves the formation of drug immune complexes that attached to the cell surface and can result in acute haemolysis with haemoglobinuria and renal failure. Severe haemolytic episodes can recur even when only small doses of the drug are re-administered. The DAT is usually positive with C3, but with some drugs that seem to complex poorly with cells, IgM or IgG can be detected. The antibody only reacts with drug-coated cells.
- Drug independent antibodies.
  The drug stimulates an antibody that reacts with the red cell membrane not the drug itself. This type cannot be distinguished from warm AIHA as the cells react with anti-IgG. The serum and eluate also react with normal red cells without the drug having to be present. This type was more common when methyldopa was a widely used drug.
- Non-immunological protein adsorption
  Some cephalosporins can alter the cell membrane causing non-specific uptake of proteins including IgG and IgM, which are detectable by the DAT.

As cases of drug associated AIHA are rare in the UK, investigation of these is performed by a small number of specialist reference laboratories.

Autoantibody immune cell destruction is not confined to red cells, both autoimmune and drug associated immune destruction of platelets can also occur.

HAEMOLYSIS POST TRANSPLANTATION

There have been a large number of reported cases of haemolysis in patients after transplantation of bone marrow, stem cells or solid organs (heart/lung, liver, etc.) caused by either donor-derived antibodies, recipient-derived antibodies or non-immune mechanisms.

In bone marrow transplants (BMT), although the donor and recipient are HLA matched they may be of different ABO and Rh blood groups. In so called minor mismatches (e.g. patient group A, donor group O) the transplanted donor cells can produce antibodies to the recipient's red cells. In major mismatches the converse situation arises; the recipient can produce antibodies to the donor cells, as in an A donor and O recipient.

If this haemolysis occurs in ABO minor mis-matches it is usually between 5 –15 days post transplant, often with an abrupt onset, a rapidly falling Hb and possible renal failure as a result of the cell destruction. Anti-A or anti-B are thought to be produced by lymphocytes transfused with the bone marrow, so called 'passenger lymphocytes'. The haemolysis subsides as the patient's remaining incompatible red cells are destroyed and replaced with those of donor origin. During the haemolytic episode the DAT may be positive and the causative antibody eluted from the patient's red cells. When investigating such cases the eluate should always be tested, by IAT with A or B cells depending on the group of the recipient. Likewise, an IAT crossmatch must be performed post-transplant even if no antibodies are detected in the antibody screen. Although ABO antibodies are most commonly implicated, other antibodies of the Rh, Kidd and Lewis blood group systems have been reported.

In major ABO mis-matches the donor's red cells could be destroyed by the recipient's ABO antibodies. This might lead to the delay in the production of the donor red cells or as erythropoesis increases the residual antibodies might lyse these cells. In these cases the haemolysis is not noted until several weeks after the transplant; times of 30-100 days have been reported. The DAT is usually positive with IgG, anti-A/B being eluted from the red cells. Depleting the marrow of red cells or reducing the patient's antibody levels can reduce the likelihood of this lysis occurring.

Autoimmune haemolytic anaemia can also occur post transplant when the donor's immune cells produce antibodies directed at the donor's red cells. This phenomenon is not common, but where it does happen it is usually approximately 10-12 months post-BMT.

(*Further reading see: Haemolysis associated with transplantation; editorial in Transfusion 1998; 38: 224-228*)

INVESTIGATION AND CROSSMATCHING

Many of the patients with a positive DAT have some kind of malignancy and have been transfused. Figures from NBS Reference laboratories show that 75% of DAT positive cases referred to them are from patients who have been previously transfused and about 40-50% have alloantibodies present.

Transfusions should be avoided in these cases if other treatments are possible. If however, a transfusion is required and the antibody screen is negative, blood can be selected and crossmatched in the normal manner, even though the DAT is positive. However, in many cases the antibody screening test is positive due to the presence of free autoantibody and then additional tests need to be employed to exclude the presence of alloantibodies which may also be present with and masked by the unbound auto-antibody free in the patient's serum/plasma.

It is important to identify these alloantibodies as they are more clinically important in selecting blood for transfusion than the autoantibodies. The investigation of these cases requires the use of specialist techniques, involving adsorption of the autoantibodies onto either the patient's own red cells, auto-adsorption, or selected reagent cells, alloadsorption (further details are given below).

Alloadsorption is used if the patient has been transfused within the past 3 months, or there are insufficient patient cells available for autoadsorption. The adsorbed serum/plasma is then tested by standard methods to detect and identify any alloantibodies present. Making and testing an eluate is only performed if the patient has been transfused within the past three months, recently received a transplant, or if there is unexplained increased destruction of transfused red cells. This might be due to a haemolytic transfusion reaction rather than the underlying AIHA, or it could be a combination of the two.

Autoadsorption is a more direct way of removing autoantibodies from the serum/plasma but in practice is used less frequently than alloadsorptions as so many patients with a autoantibodies have been transfused or there are too few red cells to work with, due to the patient's underlying anaemia. This technique cannot be used if the patient has had a recent transfusion as the transfused cells, still present in the patient's circulation, might remove the alloantibody and if not detected this antibody could cause a reaction if further blood was given to the patient.

The practice of selecting blood for patients with a positive DAT and a positive antibody screen as 'the least incompatible' units of blood by virtue of reaction strength in the crossmatch is not an acceptable procedure. Autoantibodies in the patient's serum/plasma can mask alloantibodies and it is these alloantibodies that cause rapid destruction of transfused red cells, which might exacerbate rather than help the patient's condition. Therefore selection of blood for transfusion is based on the findings of adsorption tests and the adsorbed serum/plasma might have to be used for the crossmatch. Blood tested in this way is issued as being 'suitable for' rather than 'compatible'.

In cold AIHAs is it normally sufficient to perform all tests, including ABO and RhD typing strictly at 37°C, to avoid agglutination of the cells by the cold reacting IgM autoantibody. If the autoantibody is very strong it might be necessary to adsorb the antibody onto the patient's own cells, which have first been washed several times with saline at 37°C to remove the bound antibody.

ADSORPTION STUDIES

Adsorption is used to remove the autoantibody from the patient's serum/plasma so as to be able to identify any underlying alloantibodies and therefore enable antigen negative blood to be transfused to the patient. The adsorption technique can be performed using either the patient's own red cells (auto-adsorption) or those from another person (alloadsorption).

Auto-adsorption
- Auto-adsorption should not be performed if the patient has been transfused within the previous three months.
- The patient's own washed red cell sample is usually treated with ZZAP (papain-dithiothreitol) solution to elute the autoantibodies so as to make the adsorption process more effective. Chloroquine diphosphate or acid elution can also be used to treat the red cells.

- Equal volumes of the patient's plasma/plasma and treated red cells are incubated at 37°C for about 15 minutes, then centrifuged and the serum/plasma carefully aspirated.
- To remove all, or even most, of the autoantibody this process has to be done 3 or 4 times using a fresh aliquot of cells each time.
- Following auto-adsorption, the serum/plasma is investigated for the presence of an alloantibody using standard techniques.

Alloadsorption

- The object of this procedure is to adsorb the autoantibody, which reacts with all normal red cells, but leave any alloantibody in the plasma. This will of course vary dependent upon the antigen phenotypes of the selected red cells.
- An alloadsorption technique should be used if the patient has been transfused within the previous three months or there are too few red cells available for autoadsorption.
- This technique has the practical advantage of being able to use large amounts of reagent red cells and as a result the procedure is more likely to be effective.
- Normally three aliquots of papain treated red cells are selected, which between them are able to differentiate between the major blood group antigens. For example, R_1R_1, R_2R_2 and rr cells, with at least one sample being K-, Jk(a-), Jk(b-), etc.
- As above, 3 or 4 adsorption processes, each with a fresh aliquot of red cells, are usually needed to remove all, or most of the autoantibody, so that any alloantibody can be identified.
- The plasma from each of the adsorptions should then be investigated for the presence of alloantibody using standard techniques, the presence or absence of which will of course depend on the antigen phenotypes of the selected red cells.

The following table provides an example of this procedure.

Example of alloadsorption process using three selected red cell aliquots

Adsorbing red cell Rh phenotype *	Alloantibodies and autoantibodies adsorbed	Alloantibody specificities left in serum/plasma
C+c-D+E-e+ (R_1R_1)	Allo-anti-C, -D, -e	Anti-c, anti-E
C-c+D+E+e- (R_2R_2)	Allo-anti-c, -D, -E	Anti-e, anti-C
C-c+D-E-e+ (rr)	Allo-anti-c, -e	Anti-C, anti-D, anti-E

* This simplified table provides an explanation for Rh specificities only. The reactions of the other major clinically significant antibodies should also be able to be differentiated by the red cell phenotypes of the three red cell aliquots.

(See – Detecting alloantibodies in patients with autoantibodies; editorial in Transfusion 1999; 39: 6-10)

QUESTIONS - SECTION 12

1. What are the 4 main reasons for *in vivo* mediated red cell destruction?

2. What is the direct antiglobulin test used for and what are its limitations?

3. What are the main characteristics of warm AIHA?

4. What are the main characteristics of cold AIHA?

5. What are the main characteristics of PCH?

6. What are the main characteristics of drug induced / associated haemolytic anaemia?

7. Is the DAT always positive in cases of AIHA?

8. If the DAT is positive is there always increased red cell destruction?

9. Why can immune haemolysis occur after a transplant?

10. Why are alloantibodies more important than autoantibodies when crossmatching blood for a patient with AIHA?

SECTION 13

BLOOD DONATION TESTING

INTRODUCTION

The collection and processing of donated blood and components is a highly regulated process. Included in that process is the comprehensive serological and microbiological testing of every donation to ensure it is safe for clinical use and matches the patient's requirements. The Testing process is part of the overall quality system. Testing departments must comply with Good Manufacturing Practice (GMP) and are regularly (at least once every two years) audited by internal and external inspectors, i.e. from the Medicines and Healthcare Products Regulatory Authority (MHRA), to ensure compliance both with GMP and Blood Safety and Quality Regulations (BSQR). In the United Kingdom, the requirements for testing are laid down in the 'Guidelines for the Blood Transfusion Services in the United Kingdom (the 'Red Book') and the Blood Safety and Quality Regulations (2005). Similar guidelines are found in many other countries.

Testing includes the performance of mandatory tests (i.e. performed on every donation), additional tests (i.e. performed on selected donations, e.g. CMV antibody, red cell phenotyping) and discretionary tests (i.e. the testing of donations where a donor reports a possible extra risk factor, e.g. travel to a malaria endemic area).

In the UK, the mandatory tests on every donation are ABO grouping, Rh D typing and antibody screening, as well as testing for Hepatitis B surface antigen (HBsAg), antibody to Human Immunodeficiency Virus (anti-HIV1+2), antibody to Hepatitis C virus (anti-HCV) and antibody to syphilis. In addition, all donations are tested for the presence of HCV RNA using a Nucleic Acid Amplification Test (NAT) system and antibody to Human T-cell Leukaemia Virus (HTLV) antibodies by 'mini-pool' testing (see later).

For blood grouping, samples from new and existing donors are separated. For existing donors, information on their blood group and microbiology status will be on the main computer system (blood donor grouping and testing records are archived for the whole of the UK). Providing that the results for the current donation are concordant with those on record, the donation can be released. For first time donors there is no historical record, so the ABO and Rh D type must be confirmed using a more comprehensive procedure, involving two independent test runs.

The Testing Department of a Blood Centre covers a number of sections, which may be organised as independent laboratories, though under the same departmental structure. Most testing sites will have a 'Blood Grouping' section and a 'Microbiology' section. A proportion will also have a NAT section. The specialised nature of NAT testing, with its requirement for specialist equipment and facilities, means that it is more cost effective to centralise these facilities. New automated NAT technologies do away with this requirement. In England there are eight testing departments but only three NAT departments. Due to strategic re-organisation to take advantage of newer ways of working, the number of testing laboratories in England will reduce to five by 2010.

SUMMARY OF DONATION TESTING

All donations in the UK are tested for:

- ABO group and Rh D type, which are performed by sensitive automated methods (involving bar-code sample identification and computer results manipulation). These tests are designed to detect weak antigens such as A_x, weak D and partial D types. All units are further tested for Rh types (C, c, E, e) and also K. A proportion are also tested for the presence of a variety of other antigens (including M, S, s, Duffy and Kidd), which are used for transfusion (as required) to patients who have produced atypical antibodies.

- The presence of antibodies to red cell antigens, to avoid the transfusion of potent 37°C reactive atypical antibodies in donor plasma, capable of causing a minor transfusion reaction.

- Microbiology (Virology) tests to detect:
  - HBsAg (hepatitis B surface antigen).
  - HCV / anti-HCV (hepatitis C virus / antibody to hepatitis C).
  - Anti-HIV 1 and 2 (antibody to HIV).
  - A test for syphilis antibody (i.e. TPHA or similar).

BLOOD GROUPING SECTION

The 'Grouping Section' is responsible for the primary grouping of blood donations and the investigative follow up of discrepant groups. The requirements of GMP have led to all but the smallest of centres adopting some kind of automated testing system. All UK testing centres use Olympus PK test systems. This gives the advantage of:

- Positive sample identification (PSI) using bar-coded samples
- Strict adherence to defined methods using computer controlled dispensing of reagents and samples, as well as incubation time and temperature
- Reading and interpretation of the final result is by camera (or other optical device), so the whole process is free of human error.

For every test run, samples of known type must be included to confirm the correct placing and preparation of typing and red cell reagents. The instrument of choice for larger testing sites world-wide is the Olympus PK series of machines. These use special V well microplates to perform haemagglutination tests in. The wells have steps or ridges at regular intervals down the side to facilitate good discrimination between positive and negative reactions (see below). Each plate can take ten samples and each sample has up to twelve test wells, each utilising a different reagent.

Schematic representation of haemagglutination in an Olympus plate well

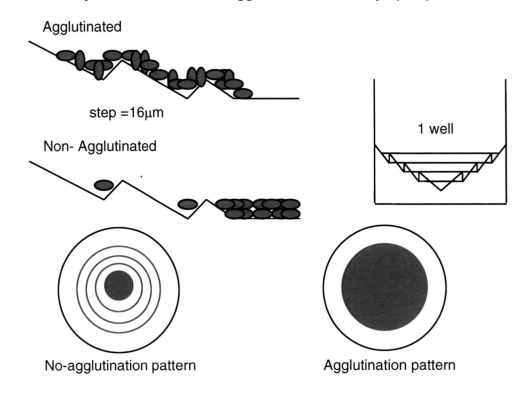

Agglutinated

step =16μm

Non- Agglutinated

1 well

No-agglutination pattern

Agglutination pattern

MANDATORY TESTING

All donations, whether from new or existing donors have a confirmatory test to identify ABO and Rh D type. Only the cell type is determined, using monoclonal anti-A, anti-B and anti-D. In Europe all typing reagents and test kits must comply with the EU Diagnostic Medical Device Directive, which is demonstrated by carrying the CE mark. In England the anti-A reagent used is selected to detect A_x cells. The anti-D used is a blended monoclonal reagent capable of detecting weak D samples and partial (variant) D types, especially DIV, DV and DVI.

An antibody screen is performed on all donations to protect against the possibility of passively transferring antibody from donation to patient, where it may react with the patient's cells or other donor red cells being transfused to the patient, if one or other carries the appropriate antigen. In the UK the 'Guidelines for the Blood Transfusion Services in the UK' (or 'Red Book') specify an antibody detection method capable of detecting anti-D at 0.5 IU/ml. In England the test is performed on the Olympus using papain treated red cells carrying the D, C, c, E, e, K and Jk^a antigens. This system will not detect antibodies that react by an antiglobulin technique or whose antigens are destroyed by enzyme treatment. This includes antibodies to the Fy^a, Fy^b, S and s antigens. The Olympus method is optimised to detect antibodies of Rh or K specificity, as these are the only ones where there is evidence of morbidity when passively acquired. In adults the dilution effect will usually be enough to render weaker antibodies non-reactive *in vivo* (the antibody screen system used for blood intended for neonates is different).

New donors are re-tested to give a second separate group result. The ABO cell group is performed against anti-A and anti-B, and the reverse group is determined by testing the donor plasma against group A_1 and B reagent red cells. The Rh D type is determined by testing against monoclonal IgM anti-D. Although there is no 'Red Book' requirement to use different typing reagents, in England the anti-A is selected to not detect A_x and the anti-D is selected to not detect DVI (see below). Therefore, new donors are tested using one set of reagents that detects A_x and DVI and a second set that does not. As such, if the donor is either A_x or DVI the resulting test discrepancy will trigger a computer query requiring further investigation.

Significance of A_x and DVI

A_x is a rare sub-group of A with weakened expression of A antigen. If not detected it will be typed as group O. If A_x red cells are transfused to a group O donor, there is a small possibility of increased red cell destruction especially if the recipient has potent IgG anti-A (see Section 3: The ABO Blood Group System). Rh DVI is the commonest of partial D types in the UK. If incorrectly typed as Rh D negative and transfused to an Rh D negative recipient it can stimulate the production of anti-D, which can have severe consequences in causing possible Haemolytic Disease of the Fetus/Newborn if the recipient is female and of child bearing age or younger (see Section 4: The Rh Blood Group System and Section 11: Haemolytic Disease of the Fetus/Newborn). It is therefore essential that A_x is detected and grouped as A, and that DVI is detected and grouped as Rh D positive. By using reagents, which do not detect A_x or DVI in the new donor test run, the resulting discrepancy will lead to further investigation, which will confirm the true type. This allows the identification of these rare cell types and provides a source of red cells as controls to confirm typing reagents are performing correctly.

Although not mandatory, all donations in the UK are typed for C, c, E, e and K, as these grouping tests can be easily performed on the Olympus, at the same time as the primary ABO / Rh D groups. The information can then be printed on the pack label. This allows hospital blood bank staff to select blood for patients with antibodies from their own stock, without having to request them from the blood centre. K typing is especially important as anti-K is the next most clinically important cause of Haemolytic Disease of the Fetus/Newborn (HDFN) after anti-D and anti-c, so most hospitals have a policy of, wherever possible, primarily selecting K- red cell units when transfusing female patients at or below child bearing age. Typing all donors gives a large database of typed donors, which is a very useful starting point when selecting red cells for recipients who may have formed antibodies to several red cell antigens. It also allows for easy matching of Rh and K phenotype to patients who are likely to have long-term dependency on red cell transfusions (see Section 8: Pre-Transfusion Testing).

High titre anti-A and/or anti-B

Passively acquired anti-A and/or anti-B, when group O blood is transfused to certain non-group O recipients, has caused morbidity and mortality. Ideally, blood of the correct type should be transfused but this may not always be possible, especially in emergency situations, when transfusing neonates, or when providing HLA or HPA matched platelet concentrates. The risk can be reduced by identifying those donors most likely to cause a reaction and labelling them 'for group O use only' (or 'for group B use only' if a group B donor has high levels of anti-A or 'for group A use only' if a group A donor has high levels of anti-B). There is no consensus on the definition of a 'dangerous' donor in these situations, or on how to identify them. Transfusion reactions of this type are almost always caused by high levels of IgG anti-A and/or anti-B in donor plasma. Lower levels of antibody may be important if large volumes of plasma or plasma containing products are transfused. In England, all donations are tested on the Olympus for high titre anti-A and/or anti-B by diluting the donor plasma to an equivalent of 1 in 56 and testing against A_2B red cells. The threshold is set to detect the strongest 5-10% of donations. It is recognised that this is an arbitrary test and is not optimised to detect IgG antibodies.

Investigation of donations with alloantibodies

Donations which give a positive antibody screen on the Olympus, or who are from donors known to have produced red cell antibodies, must be further investigated to determine if the products are safe to issue, or if the antibodies are suitable for reagent use. Weak antibodies are particularly useful as a source of material for use in external quality assurance schemes.

The Olympus antibody screen, though fairly insensitive, can detect weak Rh antibodies and most examples of anti-K. However, because it is an enzyme technique, it is prone to non-specific positive reactions. The initial investigation is to confirm whether or not any clinically significant antibody is present. This is accomplished using an antiglobulin technique. A cell (or pool of up to two cells) containing the D, C, c, E, e and K antigens may be used for testing donors (but not for neonatal use – see later). Use of modern commercial microplate capture or gel column technology is ideal for this as it can be automated using a number of bespoke or third party test systems and maintain the principle of positive sample identification (PSI) and machine read and interpreted results. If this screen test is negative then all products may be released for stock. If positive, the sample is further investigated to identify the antibody specificity and a titration test is performed to determine the antibody strength, again using an automated antiglobulin system. The 'Red Book' guidelines give the following instructions for donations with antibodies:

Positive on neat screen:	All products may be used for adult recipients only.
Positive at 1 in 10, negative at 1 in 50:	Red cells in additive solution may be used for adult recipients only, all other products not suitable for clinical use.
Positive at 1 in 50:	All products not suitable for clinical use.

For donors with strong antibodies (reactive at 1 in 50), if their plasma is not suitable or required for reagent use, the donor must be removed from the donor panel. If their plasma is suitable for use, if possible they should be encouraged to donate by plasmapheresis. Note: The above cut-off titres are used in England; slightly different ones may be used in other UK countries dependent on the techniques and validations performed.

Phenotyped Donations

Apart from the Rh phenotyping and K typing performed on all donations, a proportion of donations will be further tested to meet hospital demand for specifically typed products. These may be requested for patients with pre-formed antibodies from previous transfusions or pregnancy, or for patients undergoing long term transfusion support, to minimise the risk of them producing antibodies. The Blood Service categorises red cell antibodies into one of three classes for this purpose:

1. Cold reactive antibodies, not active at 37°C:
   - Typed units are not routinely provided.
   - Examples include anti-P_1, anti-N, anti-Le^a and anti-Le^b.

2. Antibodies active at 37°C and therefore (potentially) clinically significant, but whose corresponding antigen frequency is low enough to mean that there would be no difficulty finding compatible units on crossmatch:
   - Typed units are not routinely supplied.
   - Examples include anti-Kp^a and anti-Lu^a.

3. Antibodies active at 37°C and therefore (potentially) clinically significant, and whose corresponding antigen frequency is high enough to mean that hospitals could encounter difficulty providing sufficient compatible units by random crossmatching:
   - Typed units are supplied.
   - Examples include anti-Fy^a, anti-Fy^b, anti-Jk^a, anti-Jk^b, anti-S, anti-s and anti-M.
   - Although some examples of anti-M are cold reactive, many examples of IgG anti-M occur that frequently react by microcolumn IAT, enough to warrant inclusion of M on the list of typed antigens (see Section 10: Other Blood Group Systems).

Where monoclonal IgM reagents exist, typing of large numbers of units can be performed on the Olympus PK automated blood grouping machine (i.e. using anti-Jk^a, anti-Jk^b, anti-S and anti-M). For other types (anti-Fy^a, anti-Fy^b, anti-s), which require an antiglobulin test, typing can be performed on the automated secondary equipment, that is also used for antibody screening. Each Blood Centre holds a stock of typed units, of varying ABO groups and Rh phenotypes, sufficient to meet local demand and contribute to the national pool / stock. Depending on the ethnic mix of the population served, units of type Fy(a-b-) and S-s-U- may also be held. The later are extremely rare so when encountered, the red cells would be offered to the National Frozen Blood Bank (NFBB) for long term storage (up to ten years).

'Sickle testing' of red cells, to rule out donations heterozygous for HbS, may be required for patients suffering from haematological disorders. A solubility test in microplates can be performed on the automated equipment previously described. Donors found to be positive are confirmatory tested by a specialist laboratory to confirm the result. Heterozygote HbS positive red cells are suitable for most adult patients, however when leucodepleted, the product should have a post-filtration white cell count performed, because of the high number of filter blockages seen when filtering HbAS type donations.

Selection of products for neonatal use

Guidelines for provision of products for neonates are identified in both the 'Red book' and by the British Committee for Standards in Haematology Blood Transfusion Task Force (BCSH guidelines). These cover the selection of donors, production standards for the products and required testing. Donations used to produce neonatal products must be from donors who have had a negative microbiology screen result within the past two years. New donors and existing donors who last donated more than two years ago are excluded.

Red cells for use in massive transfusion (e.g. exchange transfusion, intrauterine or foetal transfusion, cardiac bypass surgery) must not be in an optimal additive solution. The preferred anticoagulant is citrate phosphate dextrose (CPD). Red cell products should have a haematocrit of 0.55 - 0.60 (0.70 - 0.80 for intra-uterine transfusions (IUT)) and be used within 5 days of collection (see Section 14: Blood and Blood Products).

Red cells for use in small volume transfusion (e.g. top-up to correct anaemia) may be in an optimal additive solution, e.g. Saline Adenine Glucose Mannitol (SAG-

M), and may be used up to their normal shelf life of 35 days. Ideally, to prevent waste and reduce donor exposure, one donation may be split into several aliquots (typically 6) and reserved for the same patient.

Platelets for neonatal use must come from a single donor to reduce donor exposure and attempts are made to produce these from male donors only to reduce the risk of TRALI based on the fact that the antibodies associated with TRALI are more likely to occur in women who have had children. These are produced from apheresis platelets, which may be split into aliquots (the practice in the UK) or from single unit recovered platelets.

All donations must be tested for mandatory markers. High titre ('haemolysin') anti-A and/or anti-B test positive donations must be excluded. The mandatory antibody test performed on the Olympus machine is of insufficient sensitivity for blood intended for neonatal use (due to the fact that the procedure may not detect weak examples of antibody that might be significant when transfused into the patient with a small circulation, such as a baby). A more sophisticated test, equivalent to a patient antibody screen is performed, using the automated antiglobulin procedure previously described but using a minimum of two antibody screen cells, which between them are homozygous for antigens D, C, E, c, e, M, S, s, Fy^a, Fy^b, Jk^a and Jk^b. One cell must also be positive for the K antigen. Current 'Red Book' requirements also require the presence of C^W, Kp^a and Lu^a though this is under review.

Cellular products should be tested and found negative for antibody to cytomegalovirus (CMV). Where CMV negative products are not available, leucodepletion by filtration is a suitable alternative, providing individual units have post filtration white cell counts performed to confirm filtration has been successful.

In countries where universal leucodepletion is not performed, neonatal products should be filtered. Red cell products should be tested for HbS (Note: The 'Red Book' states that 'unless the Blood Centre recommends screening is unnecessary, the component should be haemoglobin S negative'). The method described previously is suitable. Some products intended for neonatal use must be irradiated to prevent the possibility of graft versus host disease (GvHD).

MICROBIOLOGY SECTION

The 'Microbiology Section' is responsible for performing all mandatory and additional microbiology tests on blood donations. Designated departments may also offer screening for discretionary markers as a national or regional service, performing tests on behalf of several centres, to maximise resources while minimising the impact on the various departments.

Principles of Testing for Viruses

Following infection with a virus there is usually some time before the appearance of virus in detectable amounts in the blood (for those viruses transmitted by blood transfusion). Such viraemia can be detected by assays for viral antigen (protein) or for the genes of viral nucleic acid (assays generically known as nucleic acid tests or NAT; one example of this is the polymerase chain reaction or PCR). Thereafter in most individuals an immune response develops resulting first in formation of anti-viral IgM followed by IgG. All of these assays are used in detecting virus infection in donors and their utility will depend on their relative sensitivity as well as the time at which they become positive after infection.

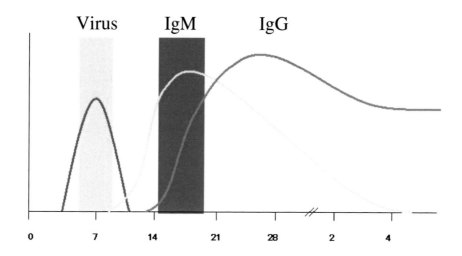

The period from infection until the first detectable marker is observed is known as the window period, during which time blood may be infective but not positive in any screening assay. The part of this time (early on) when blood is not infective is known as the eclipse period.

How infected donations may escape detection will depend on the general frequency of infection for a particular virus, the window period and the sensitivity of assays used. For those viruses for which testing is mandatory, the residual risks of blood transfusion causing infection (different from the number of reactive donations found) is very, very low, e.g. current hepatitis C testing has "cleaned" the blood donor panels so that this risk is about one in 30 million.

Donations from:	HIV		HBV		HCV	
	Per million	1 in x million	Per million	1 in x million	Per million	1 in x million
All donors	0.19	5.22	2.02	0.50	0.03	29.03
New donors	0.44	2.26	6.11	0.16	0.15	6.79
Repeat donors	0.16	6.16	1.54	0.65	0.02	46.99

Examples of the time-course for the 3 main viruses for which we undertake mandatory testing are shown below.

HIV

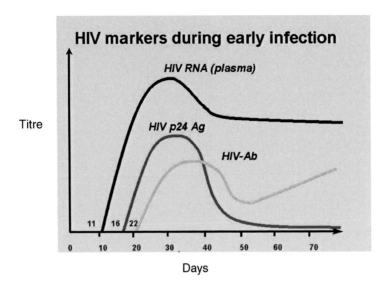

Hepatitis C

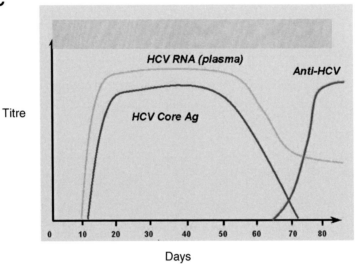

Hepatitis B
(unusual in that large amounts of excessive envelope protein is excreted from infected hepatocytes, detectable as HBsAg are produced early in the course of infection)

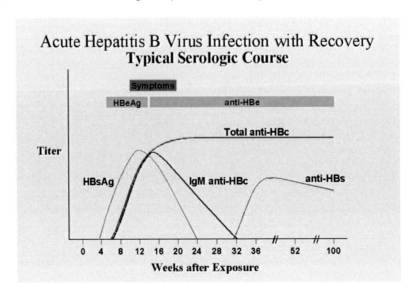

Interpretation of Results of Serologic Tests for Hepatitis B						
HBsAg	HBeAg	Anti-HBe	Anti-HBc		Anti-HBs	Interpretation
			IgG	IgM		
+	+	-	-	-	-	Incubation period
+	+	-	+	+	-	Acute hepatitis B or persistent carrier state
+	+	-	-	+	-	Persistent carrier state
+	-	+	+/-	+	-	Persistent carrier state
-	-	+	+/-	+	+	Convalescence
-	-	-	-	+	+	Recovery
-	-	-	+	-	-	Infection with hepatitis B virus without detectable HBsAg
-	-	-	-	+	-	Recovery with loss of detectable anti-HBs
-	-	-	-	-	+	Immunisation without infection, repeated exposure to antigen without infection, or recovery from infection with loss of detectable anti-HBc

PRINCIPLES OF IMMUNO-ASSAYS

All tests used in the microbiology section of Blood Centres are for the detection of antigens and/or antibodies as indicators of infection in donors. These immuno-assays use a variety of techniques to allow the detection of the resultant serological reaction. The requirements for Good Manufacturing Practice (GMP) mean there is a very high degree of automation to give positive sample identification (PSI), machine controlled process handling and computer interpretation of results, to avoid human error. In the UK, with the exception of donor syphilis screening, all tests use solid phase technology, either in a microplate format using robotic samplers and automated plate processors, or by using Abbott Prism™, a dedicated instrument for donor screening. Microplate tests use an ELISA (Enzyme Linked ImmunoSorbent Assay), while Abbott Prism™ uses microparticle CLA (Chemi-Luminescent Assay). Regardless of the instrument, the basic principle of solid phase reactions is similar.

DETECTION OF VIRAL ANTIGENS

Antibody to the antigen to be detected is coated to the solid phase (e.g. the inside of a well of a microplate) by the manufacturer. Aliquots of donor sample (serum or plasma), kit controls or external standards are added to the wells of the plate by the robotic sampler. Many modern kits include a sample diluent to be added to the wells first. This diluent changes colour when the sample aliquot is added, which allows for verification of sample addition either by visual inspection or machine reading.

1. The plate is incubated for a time period set by the manufacturer, usually at 37°C. The plate is then washed several times. If antigen is present in the samples it will bind strongly to the antibody on the solid phase. Washing removes unbound material leaving the bound antigen.

2. A conjugate reagent, consisting of antibody to the target antigen, coupled to a marker molecule, is then added. The marker molecule allows detection of the final reaction. It can be a number of substances. For ELISA it is an enzyme, most commonly horseradish peroxidase (HRP). For Abbott Prism™ it is an acridinium ester, which is chemiluminescent. Other systems may use radionuclides such as ^{125}I or fluorochromes such as fluorescein isothiocyanate (FITC). On re-incubation the conjugate will bind to any bound antigen, forming a sandwich of antibody-antigen-antibody-marker. A second wash step removes unbound conjugate so the marker will only be present if bound to the solid phase.

3. For ELISA assays, addition of chromogenic substrate such as tetramethyl benzidine (TMB) will lead to development of a colour reaction if antigen is present, which can be measured on a plate reader. This can be coupled to a computer to complete the automation step and calculate results. Abbott Prism™ uses activator solution, which causes any bound acridinium to emit a pulse of light, which is detected and converted to a reading. This can then be used by the on board computer to calculate results.

Modern assays for HBsAg detection often use monoclonal antibodies in the coating and/or the conjugate reagent. By selection of antibodies against different epitopes of the antigen it is possible to add the conjugate at the same time as the sample, thus reducing the number of wash steps. The figure below summarises the steps in detecting antigens:

Graphical representation of solid phase antigen detection assay

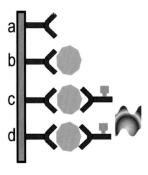

Key:
a. Solid phase coated with specific antibody.
b. If antigen is present in sample it binds to the coating antibody. Unbound material is washed away.
c. Conjugate consisting of specific antibody coupled to a marker molecule is added and binds to the bound antigen. Unbound conjugate is washed away.
d. The marker is detected by adding a reagent and measuring the signal. In ELISA this is a colour reaction. For Abbott Prism™ it is a chemiluminescence activator causing light photons to be emitted.

DETECTION OF ANTIBODIES (TO MICROBIAL ANTIGENS)

There are four basic ways of detecting antibodies. Like antigen testing, each step is marked by incubation to allow reaction to occur, followed by washing to remove un-reacted components. The final step detects the reaction by measuring the signal from the marker on the conjugate. In the case of ELISA this will be a colour reaction. Each method has its own advantages and disadvantages, either to the manufacturer, or to the user. The method used is often dependant on which manufacturer the kit is sourced from. The basic methods are summarised in the figure below.

Antiglobulin Assay

1. The solid phase is coated with specific antigens. Sample is added to the test wells along with a diluent which contains components to help neutralise non-specific factors. On incubation, specific antibody, if present, will bind strongly to the antigen. Unbound proteins are washed away.

2. The conjugate consists of a labelled anti-human globulin reagent, either anti-IgG, anti-IgM, or a mixture of both. This is added to the solid phase and on incubation will bind to any bound antibody. Unbound conjugate will be washed away.

3. The reaction is detected by adding a chromogenic substrate, allowing the colour to develop then measuring the optical density. For Abbott Prism™ the conjugate is chemiluminescent so detection is by measuring photons of light.

The advantage of the antiglobulin test is that the conjugate can be used for any antibody test system so reduces the production and quality overheads for manufacturers. The disadvantage is the relatively higher false reaction rate. All anti-HCV test systems available in the UK use the antiglobulin method, as do a number of anti-CMV kits.

Antigen Sandwich assay

1. The solid phase is coated with specific antigens. Sample is added to the test wells. In some kits a diluent is added, which allows confirmation of sample addition by changing colour. On incubation, specific antibody, if present, will bind strongly to the antigen. Unbound proteins are washed away.

2. The conjugate consists of labelled specific antigens. This is added to the solid phase and on incubation will bind to any bound antibody. Unbound conjugate will be washed away.

3. The reaction is detected by adding a chromogenic substrate, allowing the colour to develop then measuring the optical density. For Abbott Prism™, the conjugate is chemiluminescent so detection is by measuring photons of light.

The advantage of the antigen sandwich is that it is highly specific and will detect either IgG or IgM antibodies. The disadvantage is that individual conjugates must be made for each antibody to be detected and this is only cost effective for mass production. Most anti-HIV1/2 and many anti-HTLV1/2 tests use the sandwich method.

Competitive Immuno-assay

1. The solid phase is coated with specific antigens. Sample is added to the test wells along with the conjugate, which is labelled antibody of the same specificity as the antibody to be detected. For example, if the test is for CMV antibody, the conjugate is labelled anti-CMV. On incubation, specific antibody in the test sample, if present, will bind to the antigens on the solid phase. On washing, unbound proteins, including the conjugate are washed away. If specific antibody is not present in the sample the conjugate antibody is able to bind to the antigens on the solid phase and are not removed on washing. The two antibodies (the one in the sample and the conjugate) have competed for the available binding sites on the antigen. The test kinetics are arranged so that antibody in the sample wins, and blocks the conjugate antibody from binding.

2. The reaction is detected by adding a chromogenic substrate, allowing the colour to develop then measuring the optical density. For Abbott Prism™, the conjugate is chemiluminescent so detection is by measuring photons of light. Unlike the other test types, the label is present in a negative reaction, which gives a colour signal. When antibody is present in the sample it partially or completely blocks conjugate binding. Strong positive reactions lead to no colour development and weaker ones to greatly reduced colour development.

The main advantage of competitive assays is their simplicity of testing, with one incubation and one wash step. They will detect both IgG and IgM antibodies. Their disadvantage is they can only detect simple antibodies such as anti-CMV. They cannot be used in complex antibody tests such as HIV1/HIV2 tests. In blood establishments competitive assays are most commonly used for detecting antibodies to CMV, HBcAg and syphilis.

Antibody Capture Immuno-assay

1. The solid phase is coated with anti-human globulin antibodies, either anti-IgG, anti-IgM or a mixture of both. On incubation any antibody of the correct immunoglobulin class(es) will bind to the solid phase. Unbound protein will be washed away.

2. The conjugate consists of labelled specific antigens. This is added to the solid phase and on incubation will bind to any bound antibody of the correct specificity. Unbound conjugate will be washed away.

3. The reaction is detected by adding a chromogenic substrate, allowing the colour to develop then measuring the optical density. No Abbott Prism™ assay uses this method.

The advantages are as for the antiglobulin method, as manufacturers can use the same base plate, wash solution and substrate for many different assays. The major disadvantage is that the sensitivity in early sero-converters is poor. As there are relatively few specific antibody molecules in the plasma in this phase of the infection, most of the bound antibody molecules will be of different specificities giving only a weak signal. Some manufacturers improve sensitivity for early sero-converters by including specific antigens on the solid phase to give an antigen capture element, though this rules out the main advantage. One such antibody capture / antigen sandwich combi-test is used extensively for screening antenatal samples for syphilis antibodies and is the current test of choice for alternative testing of donations from donors who give false positive results by TpHA.

Graphical summary of antibody detection methods

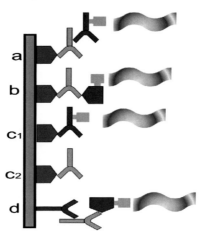

Key:

a. Antiglobulin assay:
Specific antibody binds to the antigen on the solid phase. Conjugate antiglobulin attaches to the bound antibody, allowing a signal to be detected.

b. Antigen Sandwich assay:
Specific antibody binds to the antigen on the solid phase. Conjugate antigen attaches to the bound antibody, allowing a signal to be detected.

c. Competitive assay:
In a negative test (C1) the conjugate antibody binds directly to the antigen on the solid phase, allowing a signal to be detected. In a positive test (C2) specific antibody binds to the antigen and blocks conjugate from binding. No or little signal is detected.

d. Antibody capture:
Antibodies of any specificity bind to the antiglobulin on the solid phase. Conjugate antigen attaches only to its specific antibody, allowing a signal to be detected.

Particle Agglutination assays

Particle agglutination assays use simple particles such as activated carbon or latex as the carrier. When antigen coated particles are mixed with serum or plasma and gently rocked, the particles will clump (agglutination) if specific antibody is present, while the particles remain in suspension if antibody is not present. Similarly, antibody coated particles may be used to detect antigen. They are quick and easy to perform, and are frequently used for rapid sero-diagnosis and sub-typing of bacterial infections in patients. However, they are not readily amenable to automation and are relatively insensitive so do not play a major role in donation screening in the UK.

The Rapid Plasma Reagin (RPR) test is a carbon-based test for reaginic antibodies indicative of syphilis infection and has been used for screening blood donations for many years. However, a high rate of false positives and poor specificity in primary infection have led to it falling out of favour in most European countries.

Haemagglutination assays

Haemagglutination assays are particle assays that use animal red cells as the carrier particle. Although it is possible to use human red cells, the relatively high frequency of the presence of cold agglutinins, such as anti-H and anti-I, means that there will be a large number of non-specific reactions. A number of animal red cells have been used, but the animal of choice is chicks. Chick red cells are readily available, are nucleated so settle rapidly and in the western world there is a low rate of non-specific reactions. It is easy to incorporate antigens into red cell membranes to allow detection of antibody. Such assays are called passive haemagglutination assays (PHA), because the red cells are carrying non-native antigens. It is also possible to detect antigen by incorporating specific antibodies into the red cell membrane. Such antigen detection tests are called reverse passive haemagglutination assays (RPHA). When mixed with sample serum or plasma in a U-well microplate the cells settle into a tight button at the bottom. If antibody is present in the sample (or antigen in a RPHA test) then the cells agglutinate and form a diffuse carpet of red cells across the bottom of the plate. The settling patterns for negative and positive reactions are very distinctive in appearance and easily read by eye. They look similar to the reaction patterns obtained on Olympus PK grouping machines (see above). If performed in U-well microplates the test can be automated, with sample and reagent diluent and cells being added by robotic sampler, and the completed tests read by scanning microplate readers attached to computers with data reduction software. They can also be performed on the Olympus instruments, which are designed for haemagglutination assays.

A number of assays have been used within the Blood Services, though many have now been superseded by more sensitive EIA methods. These include TpHA (*T.pallidum* haemagglutination assay), HBsAg, anti-HBc, anti-HBs and anti-CMV. In the UK, TpHA performed on Olympus is the method of choice for screening blood donors for antibodies to syphilis. For antenatal samples, a more sensitive EIA test is preferred.

One innovative Japanese company (Fujerebio Inc) have produced a range of assays based on a gelatin particle, which has a similar size and density as chick red cells and behaves in a similar way. This range of tests includes TpPA (*T.pallidum* particle haemagglutination assay), including a version for Olympus, anti-HIV1, anti-HIV1/2, anti-HTLV1, anti-CMV, anti-HCV (Latin American market only). Apart from the pastel colours of the particles, the tests are performed and interpreted in exactly the same way as for haemagglutination tests. TpPA is used on Olympus in a number of English sites for donation screening.

Selection of kits

There are many manufacturers who make test kits. Some are more sensitive than others, and many are not suitable for screening blood donors. The requirements of assays for screening blood donors, with an expectation of very few genuine positive results, may differ from the requirements for patient testing. In England, kit selection is made by the Kit Evaluation Group (KEG), made up of representatives of the NBS and the Health Protection Agency (HPA). There are also representatives of the Scottish, Welsh and Irish blood services. KEG produce a formal list of all kits approved for use in donor screening within the UK. Only approved kits from this list may be used. It is important to note that the KEG list is not a formal licensing system. In the EU this is covered by the IVD Directive. All kits must be CE marked. The KEG list performs the function of a customer suitability assessment and aids in procurement of kits to defined performance parameters and helps in agreeing contracts with suppliers. It is not an endorsement of any particular kit.

When a manufacturer approaches KEG, a formal evaluation of a new or updated kit may be agreed. The HPA will perform extensive sensitivity testing using sero-conversion panels, reference panels and other samples with previously defined performance. The National Blood Service perform specificity and performance testing of at least 2,000 tests using two different lot numbers of kit. The testing is performed in a routine laboratory, which also assesses the performance of the kit, including presentation, reagent preparation and ease of performance. If a kit meets the KEG requirements for sensitivity, specificity and performance it will be added to the list. If a contract is awarded, the performance of the kit will be regularly reviewed to ensure standards of performance do not drop. If a kit's performance deteriorates over a sustained period, or it fails to match performance of newly emerging kits, it may be removed from the list.

For Scotland and Northern Ireland a similar group to KEG known as the Microbiology Test Evaluation Group (MTEG) exists. It works closely with KEG.

Batch Pre-Acceptance Testing (BPAT)

Part of the contractual arrangement with any kit supplier will be agreement of a BPAT system. This consists, in England of two parts.

1. Lot Release Test (LRT)

Prior to shipment of any new lots to testing departments, a kit will be sent to the National Transfusion Microbiology Reference Laboratory, an independent department within the National Blood Service responsible for all reference and evaluation work. They test each lot of kit against a panel of well-characterised samples selected for their performance in a given type of kit. If satisfactory a Lot Release Certificate will be issued and registered on the NBS intranet for access by Testing departments receiving consignments of that lot. If unsatisfactory, the lot will be referred back to the supplier for corrective action.

2. Delivery Acceptance Test (DAT)

Each delivery of any given lot number will be assessed by the receiving department to ensure that there has been no performance deterioration during transit of the consignment. Only if this test is satisfactory may the delivery of kit be released for routine use. If the DAT fails, then the delivery will be quarantined pending further enquiry and the supplier notified.

Monitoring of kit performance

It is an essential part of GMP that performance of testing equipment, including assays, is monitored. The 'Red Book' guidelines lay down minimum standards and define controls. For each assay performed an independent working standard is required. Defined standards are:

- HBsAg 0.2 IU/ml
- anti-HIV1
- anti-HCV
- anti-HTLV1

In the UK, these are available from the National Institute of Biological Standards and Control (NIBSC).

- anti-syphilis QC1 for ELISA tests
- anti-syphilis QC2 for TpHA/TpPA tests
- anti-CMV

In the UK, these are available from the HPA central QA laboratory.

These standards are used as working or 'go/no-go' standards. The appropriate standard is included in every batch of tests (every plate for EIA tests, every run for Abbott Prism™) and must be clearly positive for the batch of tests to be valid. The HBsAg standard is set at the currently acceptable sensitivity level, standardised against the WHO standard for HBsAg, sub-type Ad. Although the 'Red Book' requirement is O.2 IU/ml, the actual standard is 0.05 IU/ml a level easily achieved with modern test kits and likely to be the new requirement next time the Guidelines are reviewed. There are no international units defined for antibody standards. The working standards are dilutions of strong antibodies characterised and diluted to give activity between 2 and 5 times the assay cut-off, a level agreed to be optimum for performance monitoring. Standards for anti-HIV2 and HIV p24 antigen are also available. Although used in LRT, these are not considered necessary for routine test monitoring as it is thought highly unlikely that one component of an assay would deteriorate independently of the others.

Statistical Process Monitoring (SPM)

SPM is a way of trending performance by plotting the sample/cut-off ratios of the independent standards on a chart. Although it is possible to perform manually, it is best performed using software designed for the purpose. A number of data reduction packages include Levey-Jennings plots which serve the purpose. The plot includes the moving mean value and upper and lower control limits at mean ± 3 standard deviations. Plotted values should follow a random pattern above and below the mean line. Trending involves looking for out of control conditions (these will be identified automatically by the software) and uses the 'rule of 7':

- points above the upper control limit
- points below the lower control limit
- a series of seven consecutive points above the mean
- a series of seven consecutive points below the mean
- a series of seven consecutive points ascending
- a series of seven consecutive points descending

Out of control conditions are not of themselves reason to fail a batch of tests providing the normal manufacturer's QC requirements have been met and the working standard is positive. The point of SPM is to allow investigation of trends which may be due to sub-optimal testing conditions:

- Equipment needs servicing
- Incubators and washers not at correct settings
- Reader filters dirty
- Working standard has deteriorated and needs replacing
- Lot to lot variation of kits

Understanding why an assay's SPM is out of control allows for corrective and preventative measures to be taken before assay failure occurs.

MANDATORY TESTING

Mandatory tests are those tests which must be performed on every donation of blood or blood products, regardless of how frequently the donor donates. The actual test requirements differ from country to country but as a minimum include testing for HBsAg, anti-HIV1+2 (including sub-type O), anti-HCV and anti-*T.pallidum*. Some countries also require anti-HBc, anti-HTLV1 and ALT. With modern hepatitis assays the benefit of performing anti-HBc and ALT on all donations is debatable.

In the United Kingdom, the routine donation testing laboratory performs HBsAg test (minimum sensitivity 0.2IU/ml), anti-HIV1+2 (enhanced test also detecting HIV p24 antigen) and anti-HCV. In most laboratories the syphilis test is TpHA or TpPA, performed on the Olympus blood grouping analyser (see section on blood grouping).

Although a HTLV1+2 antibody test is mandatory, different testing arrangements are in force (see section on NAT).

Handling of reactive donations

Blood donors are highly selected so the expectation in the EU is that the incidence of genuinely infected donors is very low. Nevertheless, all immuno-assay tests give rise to non specific reactions and strategies must be in place to deal with the donations and manage the donors. In the UK, the algorithms for this are clearly laid down in the 'Red Book' guidelines.

a. Initial reactive samples:

The donations of samples that are screen reactive on the first test are placed on hold pending investigation. It is a requirement of 'Red Book' and most manufacturers that the test be repeated in duplicate. Only if both replicates are clearly negative may the products be released for clinical use. If one or both of the replicates give a positive value then the products must be clearly labelled 'Not for Transfusion' and disposed of with a secure audit trail. The donor's record (computerised or manual) must be withdrawn so the donor is not called to give further donations until follow up investigation is complete.

b. Samples from repeatable reactive donations:

These must be referred to an accredited reference laboratory for complete investigation to determine whether the donor is genuinely infected or the reaction is non specific. Both the NBS and SNBTS have their own specialist reference departments which are independent of routine testing laboratories. The actual process of confirmation of reaction will differ depending on the implicated infective agent. Both follow a logical algorithmic approach. This will include:

- Alternative manufacturer's EIAs for the marker (including antigen neutralisation)
- Alternative assay types (simple/rapid assays, blot assays, line assays)
- Testing for different markers (anti-HBc, anti-HBc IgM, HBeAg, anti-HBe, HIV p24)
- Direct detection of infectious agent (NAT)

The reference laboratory for the NBS is the National Transfusion Microbiology Reference Laboratory (NTMRL). Following this approach, >70% of repeat reactive samples are found to be negative by the alternative EIAs and >99% of samples have a final conclusion.

c. Confirmed positive donations

When a repeat reactive donation is confirmed as infectious, the donor record must be marked 'Permanent exclusion risk – not to be bled for clinical use' or equivalent. It is the policy of most UK centres not to bleed such donors but some may have rare profiles (anti-HBc IgM positive, HBeAg positive, HIV p24 positive), which are particularly valuable for making standards and controls or for using in External Quality Assurance Schemes. If such donations are bled, great care must be taken to protect the staff and keep the products segregated from products and donations destined for clinical use. Donors must be contacted and counselled. Questioning will include life style and risk factors to try to identify the source of the infection. A follow-up sample will be taken and referred to the reference laboratory. The donor will also be referred to an appropriate specialist physician who will assess and provide for their future health care needs.

d. Reference negative donors

A follow-up sample is taken not less than 12-weeks after the index donation. This sample is tested at the local testing department for all mandatory markers and is referred to the reference laboratory, whether or not it is repeat reactive. If the reference result is the same as the initial one, then the donor record can be flagged 'False positive – for alternative testing', by the specific marker investigated only. Alternative testing is a system introduced in England to manage donors with non specific reactions and allow such donors to donate. It requires two negative reference results over a minimum time of 12-weeks, to make sure the donor was not in the early stages of infection at the index donation. Once the donor is reinstated, any donation given can be released immediately if the screening result is negative. If positive, the donation is quarantined until the sample can be tested by an alternative assay approved for testing blood donors by KEG. The most convenient way to manage this is to swap samples between testing centres that use different assays (e.g. between a Abbott Prism™ and ELISA site). If negative by the alternative assay, the donation can be released. If reactive the donor will be retired from the donor panel.

CMV ANTIBODY TESTING

In the UK, 43-50% of blood donors will be sero-positive for CMV. Although many countries rely on leuco-reduction methods to protect against this infection, the fact that the level of protection in certain diseases is controversial means that UK blood centres still prefer CMV antibody testing, universal leucodepletion notwithstanding. Tests of choice will detect IgM as well as IgG immunoglobulin classes, to increase detection in early sero-converters. About one third of donations are tested each day. Donors previously found to be CMV antibody positive will not be selected. Selection criteria will be driven by product stock requirements but will be specially targeted to optimise testing of platelets and fresh red cells for neonatal use. A stock of platelet concentrates for adult and neonatal use, and red cells for adult, neonatal (fresh for exchange and similar procedures) and neonatal (for top up) will be kept (see Section 14: Blood and Blood Products). These are available to hospitals on demand (i.e. 'off-the-shelf'). Products issued as suitable for neonates will automatically be selected on the basis of a negative CMV antibody test. Products can only be issued on the basis of a test on the current donation. Historical results may only be used for targeting selection of donations for testing.

DISCRETIONARY TESTING

Discretionary testing is the extra testing required to allow donors who have been exposed to specific infection risks to donate. Without testing they would need to be either temporarily or permanently deferred from donating. It is used to increase the red cell supply and increase donor satisfaction. Where mandatory testing is used to screen infected donors out, discretionary testing is used to screen non-infected donors in. The NBS has a centralised testing function to maximise kit utilisation of this relatively small number testing programme. Red cells and frozen plasma products from donations requiring discretionary testing are held in quarantine until the results are available. Platelet concentrates are not made from these donations because of the turnaround time of the testing system. The NBS rules of testing are governed both by national regulations and European Union directives, covered in UK law by BSQR..

1. Malaria is by far the commonest reason for discretionary testing as travel to and from endemic areas is prevalent. Testing is by antibody EIA.
    *   Donors who have visited an endemic area may be bled 6 months after their return provided an antibody test is performed. They may donate normally after 12 months, even without an antibody test.
    *   Donors who have been continuously resident in an endemic area for more than 6 months may donate 6 months after their return or last exposure provided an antibody test is performed. Without an antibody test they can never donate.
    *   Donors who have had confirmed malaria or an undiagnosed febrile illness after returning from an endemic area are deferred from donation for 3 years. If they re-visit an endemic area within the 3 years then they are deferred for a further 3 years from their return. After 3 years they may donate provided an antibody test is performed.
    *   Donors who have received a blood transfusion in an endemic area before 1980 may donate provided an antibody test is performed. Donors who have received transfusions anywhere in the World after 1980 are debarred from donating within the UK.

2. Chaga's disease is specific to Southern and Central America. It is caused by *Trypanosoma cruzi* which is spread by triatomine bugs. Cities are not generally a risk area as they are not an environment favoured by the bugs. Rural farming and subsistence areas are the favoured environment. By introducing antibody tests, countries such as Argentina, have virtually eradicated post-transfusion *T cruzi* infection. In countries that have not introduced screening, transfusion of infected blood may account for up to 40% of all cases. In England:

    *   Donors who have visited a rural subsistence/farming area for more than 4 weeks continuously may be bled 6 months after return provided an antibody test is performed. Without a test they may never be bled.
    *   Donors who have received a blood transfusion in an endemic area before 1980 may donate provided an antibody test is performed.

- Donors who were born in, or whose mothers were born in an endemic area may donate 6 months after return provided an antibody test is performed. Without a test they may never be bled.

Donors in malaria or *T cruzi* categories who cannot be bled may donate plasma for fractionation only, 6 months after exposure. In the UK such donors are not bled because source plasma for fractionation is obtained outside the UK.

3. 'Piercers' are donors who may be at increased risk of hepatitis B infection because they have undergone a procedure which may use inadequately sterilised instruments:

- Body piercing
- Tattoos (including semi-permanent and permanent make up).
- Acupuncture, unless by an approved practitioner.

Such donors may donate after 6 months provided they undergo anti-HBc testing. If positive a quantitative anti-HBs test is performed and products may be used only if this is positive at greater that 100 IU/l. Donors may donate normally after 12 months.

More detailed guidance on this area is given in the A-Z guide available on: http://www.transfusionguidelines.org.uk

NUCLEIC ACID AMPLIFICATION TECHNOLOGY (NAT) TESTING

NAT testing is used for the direct detection of virus by specific nucleic acid amplification. Its use has in some ways revolutionised the screening of donated blood for infectious agents by introducing a technology that can detect infection significantly earlier in the window period of infection than conventional serological means. The actual benefit in the window period reduction will depend on the organism; the longer the window period, the more the theoretical benefit in performing NAT testing. There is no regulatory requirement in the UK to perform NAT testing on individual donations. The driving force for introducing NAT testing is the European Pharmacopoeia which requires start pools for manufacturing medicinal products to be tested for HCV RNA by a validated method. The initial instruction from the European Committee on Proprietary Medicines (ECPM) followed a number of outbreaks of HCV infection in recipients of blood products which had been made from anti-HCV negative donations.

However, as a start pool can contain the plasma from 10,000 – 40,000 donations, it was considered that even in a low risk population, the chances of detecting an infected pool was high and this would place an unacceptable financial burden on the blood services due to the cost of disposing of, and replacing, such large volumes of plasma. A better system is to screen the individual donations and exclude positive plasma from entering the pool in the first place.

From this premise, modern donor NAT testing systems have developed. While HCV RNA detection is the only requirement in the UK, a number of countries, including Scotland and Northern Ireland have extended their programmes to include HIV RNA and even HBV DNA. However, the kit currently in use in England does include HIV so this is performed regardless of the requirement. When fully automated NAT systems are introduced late in 2009 HBV DNA will be added to the test panel though its benefit in pools of 24 is doubtful.

Sample pooling

To test individual donations by a NAT method is prohibitively expensive, not just in reagents and test kits, but in the specialised equipment and facilities, as well as the highly trained staff that are required to perform the test. The sensitivity of NAT tests means that it is possible to test pooled samples and still achieve the required sensitivity, thus significantly reducing the workload and the cost of the NAT programme. The 'Red Book' guidelines currently require a NAT system for HCV RNA be able to detect 5,000 IU/ml in a single donation. For a pool of 50 samples this requires a sensitivity of 100 IU/ml and in a pool of 100 samples, a sensitivity of 50 IU/ml. Pool sizes in the England are currently 48 samples (up to 96 in Scotland who use a more sensitive assay) as this fits neatly into a microplate format and is easily automated. The whole system is controlled by specialised pool management software (PMS), which interfaces with the pooling robot and resolves results down to the individual donation. If a pool is negative, then all 48 donations may be released. If positive, then all 48 donations must be quarantined while further investigation is carried out, including repeat testing of the pool. The pool size will reduce to 24 when new technology is introduced late in 2009. This will also do away with the need for specialised facilities as these instruments will fit into a routine testing laboratory.

TYPES OF NAT TEST

Polymerase Chain Reaction (PCR)

PCR is the commonest NAT test, and seen by some as the 'gold standard'. There are four basic steps to the method:

1. Extraction:
   This step is used to extract and concentrate nucleic acid from sample. It will extract all nucleic acids present, both DNA and RNA.

2. Reverse transcription:
   As PCR only amplifies DNA, when looking for RNA viruses such as HCV and HIV, this step is required to make a DNA copy of the RNA using the enzyme reverse transcriptase. This type of assay is called rtPCR. When looking for DNA viruses such as HBV this step is not required.

3. Amplification:
   The extracted DNA is heated to separate the two strands then cooled. A replicating enzyme such as *taq* polymerase is added along with a supply of bases and primer sequences specific to the virus(es) under investigation. This causes a copy of the two DNA strands to be made, doubling the concentration of specific DNA. This cycle is repeated several times. After 30 cycles there is over a million-fold increase in specific DNA.

4. Detection:
   A specific viral DNA sequence is tagged with a marker and used for detection. This probe binds to the amplified viral DNA, if present, and allows detection of the reaction. For blood screening, the favoured probe is HRP, which is used to produce a colour reaction just like in EIA tests.

Advantages:
There are a number of commercial sources for PCR equipment and reagents. This allows different companies to be used for the extraction and amplification steps, which may allow selection of the most efficient reagents and equipment for each step.

Disadvantages:
If using different suppliers for each step it can be challenging to get their equipment to interface with each other. Because PCR (or any other amplification method) is so sensitive it is very vulnerable to contamination with extraneous DNA. Special clean rooms are required for key steps like the reagent preparation and amplification steps.

Transcription Mediated Amplification (TMA)

TMA is similar to PCR and has the same basic steps, but they are all built into the assay, including reverse transcription so there is no need for separate equipment for each step. There is one major commercial system in widespread use (Chiron) which performs the whole procedure in one tube.

1. Sample preparation:
   Sample plasma is treated with detergent to disrupt viral envelope and solubilise viral DNA/RNA. Capture oligonucleotides, highly homologous to the highly conserved regions of the target viral nucleic acid, are added and hybridise with any viral nucleic acid present and attaches it to a magnetic bead which can be used in rapid washing and separation procedures.

2. Amplification:
   A reverse transcriptase is used to form a DNA copy of the viral RNA. A second enzyme, an RNA polymerase acts on the DNA template (including that from DNA viruses) to produce multiple copies of RNA amplicon. A billion-fold amplification is claimed in one hour.

3. Detection:
   This is by Hybridisation Protection Assay (HPA). Single stranded probes, complementary to the amplicon and labelled with acridinium, are added and hybridise with any specific viral RNA present. Reagent is added which inactivates the label on non-hybridised probe. Hybridisation protects the label from this step. The final signal is measured by a luminometer.

Advantages:
All of the reaction takes place in one tube, which makes it easier to handle and only needs clean room facilities for reagent preparation. No separate step is required for DNA viruses. Use of different acridinium esters for sample probe and the internal control (added to every test or calibrator to ensure correct performance, and lack of inhibitory activity in any amplification method, including PCR), allows for simultaneous detection of both sample and internal control, reducing reading time. TMA can be multiplexed so more than one virus can be detected at once. Currently, Chiron have a duplex assay to detect both HIV1 and HCV simultaneously, which is widely used in the USA and Europe, and they have also released a triplex assay, which adds HBV to the repertoire. A confirmatory test to allow assignment of the correct virus for a screen reactive sample is included in the kit.

Disadvantages:
Manual TMA is very labour intensive, requiring staff to be highly trained. One member of staff needs to follow the whole process through, which is quite stressful. Use of

different members of staff for different portions of the assay has led to higher failure rates. To address this, Chiron have developed an instrument (Tigris), which is able to perform the whole process in a fully automated GMP compliant system. It can perform up to 1000 tests (pools or singleton samples) in a single 12-hour shift.

Resolution of positive pools to individual donations

When a pool is confirmed positive, the individual donation responsible must be identified. This allows the remaining units to be released and the infected donation and donor to be handled appropriately. The English system uses a mini-pool approach. When the 48 samples that make a pool are sampled, an archive sample is also taken and stored in a deep well microplate to give a sample grid of 6 rows (1-6) and 8 columns (A-H). The archive rack from the positive pool, under control of the PMS software, is placed back on the robotic sampler and 14 mini-pools constructed, 6 pools from the rows, 8 from the columns. These are then tested and plotted against a grid. Where the positive row and column intersect, that sample is the positive one (see below).

Resolution by mini-pool

	A	B	C	D	E	F	G	H	Result
6									-
5				■					+
4									-
3									-
2									-
1									-
Result	-	-	-	+	-	-	-	-	

This strategy obviates the need to test all 48 samples individually. A similar strategy can be used for pool sizes of 24 giving cross-pools of 3 and 8. For pool sizes below this, it is easier to test the individual constituent samples of the pool. Of the 14 mini-pools, D and 5 are positive, showing the sample in D5 to be the responsible one. The PMS software can identify the individual sample stored in this well.

HEPATITIS C VIRUS

Using current assays, HCV antibody is detected about 70 days after infection, giving a long window period when screening tests would be negative but the donor potentially infectious. NAT testing will detect viral RNA in infected donors in as little as 10 days, giving a substantial reduction of the window period. Analysis of the residual risk of infection in England suggested that up to 10 antibody negative RNA positive donations per annum would occur. In fact, after more than 10 years of screening the annual detection rate is running at less than 10% of that predicted. The availability of a HCV antigen test which gives similar levels of detection as pooled NAT testing is now available and combi-assays detecting both HCV antigen and anti-HCV are also on the market. Nevertheless, the UK government has decided that NAT testing for HCV RNA must remain.

HUMAN IMMUNODEFICIENCY VIRUS

Antibody is detected about 40 days after infection. HIV RNA is detectable after 15-20 days. The reduction in the window period is less dramatic than that for HCV but nevertheless at least one documented case of post transfusion HIV infection in England would have been prevented had it been in use. Some countries routinely perform pooled NAT screening for HIV1, some by design, others because they use the commercial TMA for HCV RNA and it includes HIV1 in the screening test. Figures in the UK have found the incidence of RNA positive antibody negative donations to be less than 1/1,000,000. HIV Ag is detectable by 20 days so the use of combined antibody/antigen tests casts further doubt on the usefulness for HIV NAT screening. Nevertheless its use has expanded because HCV only NAT tests are being withdrawn from the market in favour of duplex and triplex test systems.

HEPATITIS B VIRUS

HBV DNA detection has been controversial because of its relative lack of sensitivity compared to the latest, very sensitive HBsAg screening assays. Nevertheless, Chiron claim detection of HBV RNA 13 days before HBsAg detection by a sensitive assay in their Triplex TMA NAT test. However this was on singleton samples. Testing on pools of 48 is not useful. In order to obtain any window period improvement, pools of no more than 8 samples must be used and this has considerable cost implications for the NAT screening programme.

HUMAN T CELL LEUKAEMIA VIRUS (HTLV)

Due to its very low frequency in the UK population, screening for antibodies to HTLV1/2 has not been a priority and has not been funded by the UK government. Nevertheless, cases of post transfusion HTLV infection leading to disease have been reported. In infected individuals, antibody levels are very strong which has allowed the UK to introduce a cost-effective solution. After extraction, there is sufficient residual plasma from the pooled NAT sample to allow performance of anti-HTLV1/2 tests by conventional EIA techniques. This has the benefits of introducing a screening programme for UK donors at about 2% of the price for singleton screening, with the ability to detect almost all genuinely infected donors while diluting out the majority of non-specific reactions. It is essential when introducing such a screening programme, that great care is spent on selecting the screening kit, as most do not have the sensitivity for pooled testing. The package insert for the Abbott Prism™ HTLV test, specifically excludes testing of pools.

BACTERIA

Blood donations are also on rare occasions contaminated by bacteria either from the donor's blood, or more usually by skin contaminants. This may be, and is, being addressed by improved skin cleansing at donor sessions and by diverting the first few millilitres of blood away from the donation pack. Despite this a few donations are contaminated with bacteria and can grow in blood (unlike viruses) particularly at warmer temperatures such as the 22°C used for platelet storage. It is intended that all platelets will be tested for bacteria but there is a problem in that usually very low levels are present in any contaminated donation at the time of donating and these will multiply at different rates depending on the bacterial species. Hence, how effective assays are at detecting bacteria depends on the volume sampled and when the sample is taken; the later the better but the longer the delay the greater the reduction in product shelf-life. There are a variety of assays that could be used but most are only just sensitive enough to detect bacterial contamination at a level that begins to cause reactions if transfused (about 10,000 bacteria per ml).

The most sensitive assays currently available are based on culture methods and are able to detect as low as one bacterium in the tested volume. Two commercial culture assays are currently in use in the UK. The BactALERT™ assay can detect both anaerobic and aerobic bacteria (separately) and depends on a dye colour change as a result of the change to acid pH in the cultured sample. The e-BDS™ system depends on detecting the fall on oxygen pressure in a closed system (after removal of platelets) and hence can only detect aerobic bacteria.

Surveillance data shows that most bacteria associated with platelet transfusion reactions multiply rapidly and are aerobic. Culture testing of platelets results in a reactive rate of about 1 in 200 but the rate of clinical reactions is only about one in 10,000 (it is tenfold less (i.e. 1 in 100,000) for red cells and it is not a problem for frozen components, as bacteria cease to grow in the frozen state).

An alternative approach is to subject components to pathogen inactivation treatment. Systems are now available for platelet concentrates and are under evaluation, but methods for pathogen inactivation of red cell products are still in early development.

BLOOD DONATION SAFETY – SUMMARY

The residual microbiological risk of transfusion associated disease transmission is declining with each new 'generation' of tests that are introduced. Recent estimates of the risks of a potentially infectious donation entering the blood supply in the UK (2005) are as follows:

HBV: 1 in 500,000
HIV: 1 in 5,220,000
HCV: 1 in 29,030,000
Bacteria: about 1 in 10,000

Updated figures are posted annually on the "Red Book website":
http://www.transfusionguidelines.org.uk

Only when all the tests have been completed and the results validated can donations be labelled and made available for issue. The potential risk associated with transfusion can be reduced by employing a variety of procedures, e.g.

- Improved donor selection (e.g. by the use of donor selection guidelines and confidential donor questioning).
- Improved donation testing methodologies (e.g. by use of NAT-PCR techniques).
- Quarantining of donations (e.g. for plasma products).
- Reducing inappropriate transfusions and using autologous transfusion procedures where appropriate.
- Product processing methodologies (e.g. leucodepletion, methylene blue treatment, etc.).

Product quality may be further improved by the introduction of routine viral inactivation processing of plasma products, e.g. by the use of solvent-detergent treatment, methylene-blue or psoralen / UVA treatment techniques (see Section 14: Blood and Blood Products). Due to the very small risk of transmission of vCJD by transfusion, all products manufactured for clinical use are filtered (i.e. 'leucodepleted' - using a commercial filter containing polyester fibres). Leucodepletion is used to remove white blood cells, since these are believed to be associated with the agent responsible for the transmission of vCJD. As a result, all cellular products are filtered during their preparation within the Blood Centre.

QUESTIONS - SECTION 13

1. List the mandatory tests carried out on all donations.

2. What procedures may be employed for reducing the possibility of disease transmission by transfusion?

3. What steps are taken to minimise the possible bacterial contamination of platelets?

4. Why must blood products for neonatal use have an extra red cell antibody test?

5. Why is it important to detect donors who are DVI? What Rh type should the blood pack from such a donor be labelled as?

6. What is the current sensitivity required for HBsAg screening assays used to test donors? How do we prove this level of sensitivity is achieved?

7. A hospital transfusion laboratory contacts you about a patient with anti-Kp^a in their serum and asks for typed red cells to be provided. What answer would you give the laboratory and why?

8. Give two reasons why HbS screening of red cells may be performed.

9. Briefly describe how Statistical Process Monitoring aids quality in the performance of microbiology immuno-assays.

10. What is the 'window period' of a transfusion transmitted infection?

11. Why is NAT testing done for hepatitis C but not for hepatitis B?

12. List the steps involved in the PCR test used for hepatitis C testing of blood donations and give a brief explanation of each.

13. Why might leucodepletion improve the microbiological safety of blood donations?

14. What is the current estimated risk of a patient contracting hepatitis B, HIV and hepatitis C respectively from a unit of blood in the UK?

ASSIGNMENT

Since the SHOT scheme was initiated, how many cases of transfusion transmitted HIV, HBV, HCV and bacterial infections have there been reported in the UK?

SECTION 14

BLOOD AND BLOOD PRODUCTS

Note: This section should be read in conjunction with the Handbook of Transfusion Medicine, see 'Sources of Additional Information', for reference details.

BLOOD DONATIONS - INTRODUCTION

All UK blood donors are volunteers. At the blood donor session they are asked about their health and have a finger prick haemoglobin performed. If deemed fit and healthy based on current guidelines, they are asked to sign a consent form and a donation of blood is taken. The pre-donation questioning of blood donors is based on nationally agreed 'Donor Selection' guidelines and is designed to protect the donor from donating if they are unfit to do so as well as protecting the recipient from transfusion transmissible diseases or other problems. The 'Red Book' states that a whole blood donation should have a total volume of 450ml ± 45ml of blood, collected (by weight) into 63ml of anticoagulant, however 470 ml is the more normally collected target volume. The anticoagulant is usually Citrate Phosphate Dextrose (CPD).

At the Blood Centre, the donations are processed to produce principally red cells, platelet concentrates, fresh frozen plasma (FFP) and cryoprecipitates for transfusion. Plasma for fractionation, clinical FFP and cryoprecipitate for those aged under 16, is currently obtained from non-UK donors, due to government restrictions related to the potential problem of the transfusion transmission of variant Creutzfeld-Jacob disease (vCJD). This plasma is processed by either the Bio-Products Laboratory (BPL) at Elstree (England) or the Plasma Fractionation Centre (PFC) at Edinburgh (Scotland), to be manufactured into albumin, Factor VIII and immunoglobulins (including anti-D immunoglobulin).

PREPARATION OF BLOOD COMPONENTS

The clinical demand for specific blood components has risen over the years so that all donations are now being processed into blood components. The production of blood components has been made possible by the use of large volume centrifugation techniques, the availability of sterile multiple interconnected plastic blood pack systems and sterile tube-connecting devices.

Blood components are produced in order to provide a concentrated form of a clinically effective product for the patient. This enables treatment of a specific deficiency in the patient without wasting the other components, which would be present in whole blood. Large amounts of specific products can also be administered in relatively small volumes, compared with that required if whole blood is used. Blood component production also enables the red cells, platelets and plasma to be stored at their optimal temperature and conditions and enable the components of a single donation to be used in the treatment of different patients, providing the most effective use of each unit of donated blood.

A potential disadvantage of the production and use of blood components and fractionated plasma products is the increase in the possibility of disease transmission, since the recipient is exposed to material from a larger number of donors, especially from plasma fractionation products. However, stricter and more sensitive pre-processing testing regimes, together with modifications to processing stages during production, has greatly improved the safety of these products. The introduction of universal leucodepletion (white blood cell removal) to reduce the risk of transmitting vCJD and the use of methylene blue for pathogen inactivation are such innovations.

Good Manufacturing Practice (GMP)

The processing, preparation, handling and storage of blood components is strictly controlled and GMP Guidelines must be followed at all times. Blood Centres, like pharmaceutical manufacturers are required to be licensed and regularly inspected by the Medicines and Healthcare products Regulatory Agency.

PROCESSING

Collection Packs

All blood collection packs have at least one in-line leucodepletion filter allowing the removal of white cells to be carried out during processing. As filtration is by far the most common method of leucodepletion the two words [filtration and leucodepletion] are often used interchangeably in component preparation.

There are two main configurations of multiple blood pack in common use. The type used influences what components can be produced from that donation:

a. 'Whole Blood Filter' (WBF) pack

As its name suggests this has a filter close to the main collection bag allowing leucodepletion to be carried out before separation of components. The advantage of this is that the components produced do not have to be leucodepleted separately. Blood collected in this pack type can be used for the production of red cells and frozen plasma components. The red cells are usually suspended in SAG-M from these packs but it is flexible enough to produce 'plasma reduced red cells', which are used for exchange and intrauterine transfusions. Unfortunately the filter also removes a large number of platelets along with the white cells, so this pack type is not suitable for platelet production. This type of blood pack is sometimes known as 'Top and Top'.

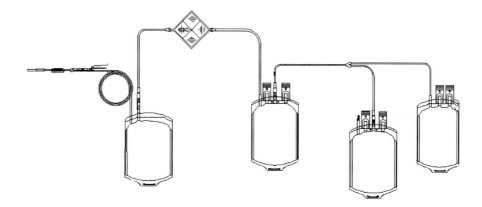

b. 'Bottom and Top' (BAT) pack

This pack type must be used if platelets are to be produced. It is distinguished from a WBF pack by the tubing coming out of the bottom and the top of the collection pack, hence the name. Separation of components is carried out before leucodepletion thus allowing platelets to be extracted. The disadvantage of this configuration is that each component must be filtered separately at the end of the process. BAT packs can be used to produce the same components as WBF packs [red cells in SAG-M and plasma] and platelets.

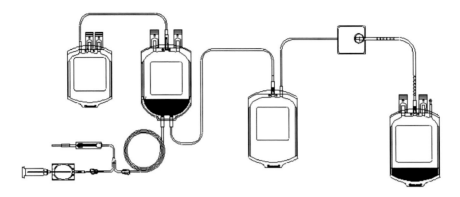

Centrifugation

Centrifugation at high force (3-4000 x g) is used to separate cellular matter from the plasma. For a WBF pack the leucodepletion will have been done before centrifugation and the red cells will be deposited at the bottom with a clear demarcation from the plasma above. BAT packs produce an extra layer on the interface called a 'buffy coat'. This layer contains most of the white cells and platelets from the donation and can be used for platelet production. Centrifugation parameters are carefully chosen to give good separation without damaging any cellular components and to maximise the amount of plasma that can be separated.

Separation

Separation of the centrifuged components is carried out using an automated press. Depending on the pack type used the plasma, red cells and buffy coat (if produced) are pressed into different bags of the multiple pack, heat sealed and detached ending up in different packs.

Platelet Pooling

The buffy coat produced when processing a BAT pack contains over 80% of the platelets from the original donation and if pooled together with other buffy coats provides an excellent starting material for platelet production.

Buffy coats (usually four) of the same ABO type are joined together using a sterile connecting device (this device 'welds' tubing together in an aseptic manner by use of a heated copper blade). A unit of plasma (or platelet additive solution) is also added to provide a storage medium for the platelets after separation. The contents of the four buffy coats are pooled into a single bag and a platelet storage bag with filter is attached. The pool is centrifuged gently to separate the red cells and white cells (which are discarded) from the platelets, which are left suspended in the plasma (or additive solution). An automated press is then used to transfer the platelets (via the filter) into the storage bag making a leucodepleted platelet pool.

Platelet pools are stored at 22°C ± 2°C and gently agitated throughout their shelf life, which is 5 days. With suitable bacterial testing the shelf life can be extended to 7 days. Extended storage of up to 7 days is possible, but bacterial testing or pathogen inactivation should be performed to mitigate for the increased risk of possible bacterial proliferation.

Automated Component Donation

Blood components can also be taken at the donors' bedside directly using machines. These allow red cell, platelet or plasma only donations to be taken with the remaining components being returned to the donor. More recent models allow two red cells units, two platelet units, two plasma units or combinations of these (e.g. one platelet and one plasma) to be taken in one donation session, depending on the particular donor.

All these machines are based on centrifugal techniques, but also rely on other technology to provide pure preparations of individual components. All machines can also directly produce leucodepleted components. For platelet products this approach has the advantage of reducing patient exposure as rather than receiving a pool of platelets recovered from four whole blood donations, one adult dose can be obtained from a single donor. Within the UK, over half of platelet donations are collected by component donation at present and this is planned to increase to eighty percent.

The ability to collect two red cell units from one donor has the potential to allow collection of more red cell units of one group in times of shortage although it should be noted that European regulations only permit the same number of donations to be collected from any one donor in each year.

BLOOD COMPONENTS PRODUCED

Specifications for all components collected in the UK are given in the Red Book (Guidelines For The Blood Transfusion Services In The United Kingdom, 7th Edition, 2005, available on http://www.transfusionguidelines.org.uk that now incorporates the requirements of The Blood Safety and Quality Regulations 2005). For most red cell components the product should now contain at least 40 g haemoglobin.

1. RED CELLS

A number of red cell products are available from stock, whereas washed red cells and reconstituted frozen red cells are available by special request. All of these products are routinely leucocyte depleted (filtered) and have a white cell count of $<5 \times 10^6$ per unit; they have a shelf life of 35 days at $4^\circ C \pm 2^\circ C$.

a. Whole blood

The 'Red Book' identifies that this should comprise 450ml ± 45ml of donor blood (collected into Citrate-Phosphate-Dextrose-Adenine (CPDA-1) anticoagulant) post-leucodepletion. As all whole blood donations are normally processed into components, whole blood is now usually available only by special request.

b. Red cells (plasma reduced)

Plasma reduced red cells are produced from whole blood that has had approximately 220ml of plasma removed following a single centrifugation technique. The packed cell volume (PCV) of the red cells is 50%-70%. Plasma reduced red cells are being phased out for all except paediatric use. This is due to the risk of TRALI associated with the transfusion of plasma and possible plasma associated infectious agents.

c. Red cells in additive solution

These are concentrated red cells that have been prepared from whole blood by the removal of nearly all of the plasma. The red cell mass is then re-suspended in a preservative solution of Saline-Adenine-Glucose-Mannitol (SAG-M), from a sterile plastic pack interconnected to the blood pack. The PCV of SAG-M red cells is 50%-70%. The advantages of producing SAG-M red cells are:

- Adenine, which is beneficial for maintaining red cell metabolism and hence survival during storage, is added to the red cells after plasma removal.
- Mannitol helps to reduce the degree of storage related haemolysis.
- Red cells suspended in SAG-M solution have a flow rate approaching that expected of whole blood.

d. Reconstituted frozen red cells

Only donations that have a rare blood group, such as Vel negative, Fy(a-b-), etc., are kept frozen, at $-80^{\circ}C$, in the UK. These are reserved for those patients who have antibodies that would react with most units of blood crossmatched. When such red cells are frozen they need to be protected in some way to prevent red cell water loss occurring due to osmotic shock, caused by the increased extracellular ion concentration produced during ice formation. Glycerol is used as the red cell cryoprotectant as it rapidly enters the red cell and binds water molecules, effectively limiting the amount of ice formation and the distribution of salts during freezing.

The glycerol has to be removed by washing when the red cells are thawed, prior to use. Thawed and washed red cells should be used as soon as possible, but can if necessary be stored at $4^{\circ}C \pm 2^{\circ}C$ for up to 5 days.

Summary of red cell blood component information

COMPONENT	CONSTITUENTS / QUALITY PARAMETERS	SHELF LIFE
WHOLE BLOOD	Volume 450ml ± 45ml (leucodepleted) Hb >40g/unit.	35 days
RED CELLS (plasma reduced)	Volume of 280ml ± 60ml. Hb >40g/unit.	35 days
RED CELLS IN SAG-M ADDITIVE SOLUTION	Volume of 280ml ± 60ml. Hb >40g/unit	35 days
SALINE WASHED RED CELLS	Locally specified volume range. Hb >40g/unit. Residual protein <0.5 g/unit.	24 hours *
THAWED - WASHED RED CELLS	Locally specified volume range. Hb ≥36g/unit. Supernatant Hb ≤2 g/unit	5 days[+] *

*   These red cell products should be used as soon as possible after preparation. If storage is unavoidable this product should be stored at $4^{\circ}C \pm 2^{\circ}C$.

[+] Use within 24 hours if red cells are suspended in saline

2. LEUCOCYTES (Granulocytes)

Leucocyte (granulocyte) blood products are used in the treatment of patients with certain types of leukaemia and other patients experiencing chronic bacterial infections or life threatening septicaemia. To be clinically effective, a dose of approximately $2x10^{10}$ cells is required, usually for a number of occasions over a few days. The leucocytes present in a unit of fresh whole blood is equivalent to approximately $1.5x10^9$ cells, therefore to provide sufficient numbers of cells, leucocyte products are prepared via a continuous flow cell separator apheresis technique. A variety of sophisticated cell separation machines are commercially available for performing this procedure, all of which employ the same basic technology.

Continuous flow cell separation makes use of the principle of differential density centrifugation to concentrate the buffy coat layer in an extracorporeal circulation whilst blood is continuously returned to the donor. The donor blood is anticoagulated and mixed with an agent to aid red cell rouleaux formation and the separation of the buffy coat. Whilst centrifugation occurs, various outlet ports, controlled by separate pumps, continuously remove the red cells and plasma components for infusion back to the donor. The technique is time consuming to perform and very expensive.

Buffy coats, separated as part of the production of pooled platelets, are used if granulocytes are not available. A method is under validation (March 2009) to produce a refined pooled buffy coat product.

Summary of leucocyte blood product information

COMPONENT	CONSTITUENTS	SHELF LIFE
GRANULOCYTES (APHERESIS)	Citrated plasma (nominal volume) with >15 x 10^9 granulocytes per unit.	24 hours *

*   Granulocyte products should be used as soon as possible after preparation. If storage is unavoidable this product should be stored at $22^{\circ}C \pm 2^{\circ}C$ for up to 24 hours.

3. PLATELET CONCENTRATES

Platelets need adequate oxygen exchange for the preservation of function and lacking this the platelets undergo anaerobic metabolism producing lactic acid which reduces the pH during storage. The platelets are irreversibly damaged when the pH reaches approximately 6.0 (or below). The storage of platelet concentrates is therefore designed to improve gaseous exchange, avoid anaerobic metabolism and therefore maintain pH levels (i.e. at between 6.4 - 7.4). The factors affecting pH and gas exchange are:

- Mixing:
  Gentle continuous mixing of platelet concentrates improves gaseous exchange through the plastic pack and reduces the amount of anaerobic metabolism, though vigorous mixing causes physical platelet damage.

- Volume / Concentration:
  Gas exchange is improved by storing a relatively small volume in a large capacity pack, increasing the surface area to volume ratio. The storage pH is maintained better when the platelet number to plasma volume ratio is optimal.

- Plastic pack:
  The specially designed plastic used for platelet storage packs is more gas permeable and therefore improves oxygen transfer with the plasma, maintaining pH.

- Temperature:
  Platelets are best stored at $22^{\circ}C \pm 2^{\circ}C$ so that they continue to metabolise glucose etc. If stored at $4^{\circ}C$ they will aggregate. Platelet concentrates can be stored for up to 5 days.

It is recommended that patients are transfused with platelets that are the same ABO group as their own, wherever possible. However, due to the relative rarity of group B and AB donors, only group O and A platelet concentrates are normally prepared. The recommended transfusion policy for platelets identifies the potential risk of transfusion ABO antibodies in the donor plasma. If an alternative ABO product has to be used due to urgency, then preferably 'lysin free' products should be selected.

Platelet concentrates – transfusion policy

Patient's ABO group	1st Choice product	2nd Choice product	3rd Choice product
O	O	A or B (lysin free)	-
A	A	B (lysin free)	O (lysin free)
B	B	A (lysin free)	O (lysin free)
AB	AB*	A or B (lysin free)	O (lysin free)

* Group AB platelets are often in short supply

Due to the presence of contaminating red cells, D negative women (of childbearing age) should be transfused with Rh D negative platelets. In addition, platelets are also prepared from CMV-antibody negative donors for use in specific immunocompromised patient groups.

a. Single unit recovered platelets

A single unit of platelet concentrate is currently prepared by separating a platelet concentrate collected by component donation techniques (see later). The resulting small volume platelet concentrate is used for patients with small blood volumes, e.g. children.

b. Buffy coat derived - pooled platelets

See above for a description of the processing of whole blood donations into platelet concentrate products (i.e. using BAT packs). Usually the platelets from 4 donations (of the same blood group) are pooled to produce 'one adult dose'.

c. Component Donation platelets

Platelets (as well as plasma or white cells) may be collected from donors using automated machines, involving an extracorporeal technique whereby the required component of blood is removed and the rest returned to the donor. A dedicated 'intermittent flow' cell separator machine is used, which is different from the ('continuous flow') method that is used for leucocyte collection. This technique enables more platelets to be collected from each donor than is possible by the conventional whole blood collection method. A platelet concentrate collected from a single donor by this method is normally expected to be equivalent to four recovered single units or one platelet pool. This method is used for the provision of HLA (Human Leucocyte Antigen) and/or HPA (Human Platelet Antigen) matched / compatible platelet donations.

Summary of platelet component information

PLATELET TYPE	CONSTITUENTS / QUALITY PARAMETERS	SHELF LIFE
BUFFY COAT DERIVED – POOLED	Volume nominally >160ml. Platelets $\geq$240 x 10^9 / pool.	5 days
COMPONENT DONATION	Volume nominally >160ml. Platelets $\geq$240 x 10^9 / unit.	5 days

(See also: 'Guidelines for platelet transfusion', see Sources of Additional Information for reference details).

PLASMA PRODUCTS

Currently pathogen inactivation is carried out on FFP and cryoprecipitate only, and is used for transfusion to all patients born after 1st January 1996.

Pathogen Inactivation of FFP (Methylene Blue)

Methylene blue is a nuclear stain used in cytology and used clinically in the treatment of methemoglobinemia. It has been used for pathogen inactivation for many years with over 2.5 million units of FFP having been treated to date in Europe. The inactivation process with methylene blue exploits it's ability to attach to the base pairs in the nucleic acid double helix. Exposure of the plasma to a controlled quantity of light (yellow spectrum, 590nm) activates the methylene blue molecules causing damage to the genetic material and disrupting viral replication and infectivity.

Although there is no accepted clinical requirement to remove excess methylene blue and breakdown products, post-processing removal filters do exist and are used in this application as the product is destined for neonates and older children.

Due to the method of action methylene blue can only be used for the pathogen inactivation of plasma. Methylene blue treatment can be carried out on fresh plasma or plasma that has been previously frozen. It is critical that plasma is leucodepleted prior to treatment as the methylene blue will be preferentially absorbed by the white cells if they are still present.

Methods of pathogen inactivation for red cells and platelets are being developed; the use of photo-inactivation using psoralens, such as amotosalen, and riboflavin for platelets appears particularly promising and is currently being validated for use.

After methylene blue treatment, the plasma can be frozen as a single unit of FFP, split into 4 smaller units for neonates, or further processed to cryoprecipitate.

a. Fresh frozen plasma (FFP)

Single unit recovered FFP

This component is prepared by removing >150ml of plasma (dependant upon the donor PCV) from a whole blood donation and rapidly freezing the plasma (i.e. to a core temperature of -30°C). FFP can also be prepared for neonatal use by splitting an FFP pack into four units, so that the final nominal volume of each pack is ~50ml. Store at -30°C or below. Once thawed FFP should be administered with minimum delay, but within 4 hours. Cryoprecipitate depleted plasma may also be produced.

Component Donation FFP

Plasma is collected as a 'by-product' of apheresis cell separator technique platelet collection as a larger volume per donor. This is useful as a way of building up stocks of AB FFP for universal use.

FFP – transfusion policy

Recipient Group	O	A	B	AB
1st choice	O*	A	B	AB***
2nd choice	A	AB***	AB***	A**
3rd choice	B	B**	A**	B**
4th choice	AB***	-	-	-

*	Group O FFP must only be given to group O patients
**	Tested and found to be negative for high-titre ABO antibodies
***	AB plasma, though haemolysin free and suitable for patients of any ABO group, is often in short supply

a. Cryoprecipitate

Initial cryoprecipitate preparation is the same as for FFP. However, once frozen, the plasma is then allowed to thaw (for up to 18 hours) at 4°C under controlled conditions. This results in a precipitate being produced which is rich in certain coagulation factors, especially Factor VIII and Fibrinogen. The precipitate is isolated and re-frozen in a small volume of autologous plasma (i.e. it goes back into solution). One unit of cryoprecipitate has a nominal volume of ~35ml and a Factor VIIIc content of >70 iu per unit. Most cryoprecipitate is pooled to make administration easier; five units usually make a pool. The quality parameters for pooled cryoprecipitate are therefore five times those of a single unit. Once thawed, FFP and cryoprecipitate must not be re-frozen and should be used immediately. If unavoidable, storage should be at ambient temperature and used within 4 hours (see also: Guidelines for the Blood Transfusion Services in the UK; see Sources of Additional Information, for reference details).

Summary of plasma product information

COMPONENT	CONSTITUENTS / QUALITY PARAMETERS	SHELF LIFE
FRESH FROZEN PLASMA (FFP)	CPD plasma (nominally >150ml), nominally separated and frozen within 8 hours of collection, with a FVIIIc concentration of >0.7 iu/ml.	2 years at -30°C or below
CRYOPRECIPITATE (POOLED)	Cryoprecipitate from five single units of CPD plasma (nominally 150-250ml), with Fibrinogen >700 mg/unit and Factor VIIIc >350 iu/unit.	2 years at -30°C or below

IRRADIATION OF BLOOD COMPONENTS

It is essential that for patients whose immune system is suppressed / immuno-compromised (e.g. neonates and bone-marrow transplant patients) that any residual white blood cells are rendered incapable of being able to multiply (in the patient's bone marrow) after transfusion. This ensures that any white cells in the blood component do not cause 'transfusion associated graft versus host disease' (TA-GvHD). Therefore, red cell, platelet and granulocyte blood components for these types of patients are gamma irradiated prior to transfusion, with a recommended minimum dose of 25 Gray (Gy). X-ray irradiation is likely to replace gamma irradiation, as it produces the same results without the security and environmental problems of using radioactive sources. See also 'Guidelines on gamma irradiation of blood components for the prevention of transfusion-associated graft-versus-host disease'; see Sources of Additional Information for reference details.

COMPONENTS FOR USE IN INTRAUTERINE / EXCHANGE TRANSFUSION OF NEONATES AND INFANTS UNDER ONE YEAR

Note: This section should be read in conjunction with 'Guidelines for administration of blood products: Transfusion of infants and neonates', see Sources of Additional Information for reference details).

Transfusion products for these purposes, as well as the mandatory donation testing and product preparation procedures described above, may also require some or all of the following, dependant upon their intended use:

General Requirements
- Prepared from a donation provided by a donor who has given a previous donation
- Tested and found to be CMV antibody negative
- Identified to be free of clinically significant red cell alloantibodies (as tested by sensitive antibody detection technique(s), equivalent to those used for the pre-transfusion testing of patients)
- Group O material should be identified to be free of high titre anti-A,B
- Leucodepleted (<5x10^6 leucocytes)

Red cells for Exchange Transfusion
In addition to the above general criteria:
- Hct between 0.50 and 0.55
- <5 days old at time of transfusion
- Gamma-irradiated prior to transfusion and used within 24 hours of irradiation.
- HbS screen negative

Red cells for Intrauterine Transfusion

Specification as for exchange transfusion (above), but haematocrit between 0.70 and 0.85. This reduces the risks associated with transfusing a larger volume.

PLASMA (FRACTIONATED) PRODUCTS

Fractionated plasma products are currently produced from non-UK derived plasma, which was introduced by the government as a precaution against the possible spread of vCJD via transfusion.

The clinical need for concentrated plasma protein fractions was the impetus to the development of large-scale fractionation methods. Basically, the method depends on the selective precipitation and subsequent extraction of plasma proteins from fresh plasma by cold alcohol. Changing the alcohol concentration, pH and temperature, precipitates different protein fractions from whole plasma. Plasma fractionation was first described by Cohn in the late 1940's.

Frozen apheresis FFP is obtained from abroad and sent to the Bio-Products Laboratory (England) or the Plasma Fractionation Centre (Scotland) for subsequent fractionation into albumin, immunoglobulin and coagulation products. The process involves the pooling of large quantities (i.e. 1000 to 1500 litres) of these individual plasma donations. All donations are individually microbiology screened for transfusion transmitted viruses prior to pooling and all donors are screened for possible infection markers.

Simplified basic plasma fractionation method

The frozen plasma is thawed to produce cryoprecipitate (used to prepare some coagulation factor concentrates), which is the first stage in the fractionation process. The remaining cryosupernatant is then treated sequentially, in the cold, with various concentrations of ethanol and buffers, to precipitate the fractions containing the different plasma proteins, which are then further purified. These purified fractions are then prepared as either freeze dried powder or stabilised solutions of known concentration, ready for use. A variety of virus inactivation processes are used to ensure that the products are viral free. The following products are produced:

a. Albumin Products

Human albumin solution (HAS) is prepared as 4.5% or 20% solutions containing approximately 45 g/l and 200 g/l concentration of albumin respectively. The solutions contain not less than 95% albumin (as a percentage of total protein), the final product being sterilised by filtration and heat treatment at 60°C for 10 hours. HAS is a ready to use solution having a storage life of 3 years at 20°C. Although it has a variety of uses, HAS is mainly used to restore plasma volume after trauma, surgery or 'shock'.

b. Immunoglobulin Products

Immunoglobulins may be prepared as two distinct types of product, dependant upon the origins of the starting plasma.

Normal Human Immunoglobulin

This product is derived from the fractionation of un-selected pooled normal plasma donations and therefore contains the immunoglobulin content reflecting the immune status of the general blood donor population. Intramuscular normal human immunoglobulin is used in the treatment of a variety of disorders and prophylactically to prevent hepatitis A infection (e.g. prior to foreign travel). Intravenous normal immunoglobulin preparations are also available which are used to treat a variety of autoimmune disorders and patients with immunodeficiency.

Specific Human Immunoglobulins

These are derived from the fractionation of pooled plasma from specifically selected donors who are known to have specific high titre antibodies, produced as a result of previous infection or active immunisation. These individual donations are initially found by random screening of blood donors or from known donor medical history. Specific human immunoglobulin preparations are used for providing passive immunisation against a variety of infections, e.g. rabies. Rh D immunoglobulin is prepared from pre-selected pooled plasma donations which contains high titre anti-D and is used in the prevention of Haemolytic Disease of the Fetus/Newborn (see also the 'Recommendations for the use of anti-D immunoglobulin for Rh prophylaxis', see Sources of Additional Information for reference details). Typical products are:

- Anti-D (immunoglobulin): 250 IU / 500 IU / 2500 IU
- Anti-Tetanus: 250 IU
- Anti-Hepatitis (B): 200 IU and 500 IU
- Anti-Varicella Zoster: 250mg
- Anti-Rabies: 250 IU

All of the above immunoglobulin preparations are given by intramuscular injection.

c. Coagulation Factors

These are produced as purified freeze-dried concentrate powders of known purity and potency. A variety of viral inactivation processes are used to ensure that the products are viral free. Typical products are:

- Factor VIII (8Y)
- High purity Factor VIII (Replenate or Liberate)
- High purity Factor IX (Replenine-VF or HIPFIX)
- Anti-Thrombin III

Other special coagulation factors (e.g. Factors VII and XI) are also available for the treatment of named patients.

STORAGE OF BLOOD AND BLOOD COMPONENTS

Red cell concentrates or red cells in SAG-M solution

Storage cabinets for red cells should comply with the British Standard BS4376 (part 1). These products should be stored at a core temperature of $4^{o}C \pm 2^{o}C$. The air temperature of the cabinet must be maintained between 2°C and 6°C and an alarm must sound if the temperature goes outside this range. An independent thermograph should record the temperature of a simulated product (i.e. a temperature probe in 100ml of water). The record charts must be stored for a minimum of 11 years. The air temperature should be indicated on the outside of the cabinet by a dial or digital display. Red cell concentrates and red cells in SAG-M solution have a shelf life of 35 days. However, SAG-M is licensed for 42 days storage and this is likely to become the norm in the near future.

Platelet concentrates

These products should be stored at 22°C ± 2°C for no more than 5 days and a continuous record kept of the storage temperature.

Fresh frozen plasma, Cryoprecipitate and Cryoprecipitate-depleted plasma

These products should be stored at a temperature of -30°C or below and kept for no more than two years from the date of preparation. Again a record chart of the storage temperature should be kept. These products contain labile coagulation factors and as such must not be allowed to thaw at any time during storage, since this will result in a dramatic loss of clotting factor activity.

Summary of the storage conditions of blood components

PRODUCT	STORAGE TIME	STORAGE TEMPERATURE	MONITORING EQUIPMENT
RED CELLS	35 days	4°C ± 2°C	Temperature recorder and alarm.
PLATELETS	5 days	22°C ± 2°C	Temperature recorder and alarm.
FFP/CRYO	2 years	Below -30°C	Temperature recorder and alarm.

Transport of blood components

Blood components and products transported between Blood Centres, Blood Banks and wards, etc., should be in a container suitable to maintain the temperature within the ranges specified above.

QUALITY MONITORING OF BLOOD COMPONENTS

For details of quality monitoring tests and the frequency with which they should be performed, see chapter 8 of the 'Guidelines for the Blood Transfusion Service in the UK' 7th Edition 2005 (see: Sources of Additional Information for reference details).

QUESTIONS - SECTION 14

1. List the storage criteria for 'red cells for transfusion'.

2. What are the advantages of producing SAG-M red cells?

3. Identify the factors that affect the pH of stored platelet concentrates.

4. Identify the additional criteria required of products intended for neonatal transfusion.

5. What are 'specific human immunoglobulins' and what are they used for?

6. Complete a table of product storage temperature and life span of the following products: red cells, platelets, FFP, cryoprecipitate and HAS.

7. Reconstituted frozen red cells are used for transfusion of what type of patient?

8. What are the principle constituents of a cryoprecipitate?

9. What are the three main categories of protein concentrate produced by fractionation of plasma?

10. What is the minimum number of granulocytes in a granulocyte concentrate and how are these produced?

SECTION 15

QUALITY

Quality is an essential aspect of laboratory work and has many definitions (see the end of this section for a glossary of definitions / terminology). If a quality approach is not adopted and errors are not addressed, then the consequences for patients and the organisation / hospital (in terms both of patient care as well as potential litigation and claims for compensation based on the Consumer Protection Act) can be far reaching. It is also recognised that quality cannot just be 'added-on' at the end of the process but has to be 'built-in' to the system of working, with the responsibility for implementing quality being that of all staff and not just the remit of specified individuals such as a 'Quality Manager'.

The recent UK Blood Safety and Quality Regulations, BSQR (2005), which are based on European legislation, also describe the Quality System requirements for both Transfusion Services and Blood Banks. Further advice on these requirements is given in documents from the Department of Health and from the Operational Impact Group (listed in the further reading Section below)

QUALITY POLICY

What 'quality' means to a laboratory should be defined within its 'quality policy'. This policy (set out by management) should identify the intentions and direction of the department with regard to quality. The management structure must be defined, be known to all, and be in a position to effectively implement both local and national policies as required. To ensure that the policy is effectively implemented a 'Quality System' needs to be in place which defines:

- Who is responsible for what
- What documentation is required
- The resource needed to run the system

To ensure that a quality system is functioning there needs to be control over how things are done and a means of gathering first hand evidence to enable a review of performance. The following areas may form part of this system:

- Document control
- Complaint reporting
- Incident reporting
- Audit trail capability

QUALITY SYSTEM

A quality system gives individuals and customers confidence that an organisation has the systems and procedures in place to produce a high quality service / product. The quality system is controlled by two main documents:

The Quality Manual

This is a managerial statement of intent, available to all staff, which defines:
- Management responsibilities
- Control of purchasing
- Documentation of procedures
- Equipment maintenance / calibration
- Product monitoring, handling, storage and tractability
- Records maintenance
- Staff training

The Document Control Policy:

This is a policy defining how documents (SOPs, forms, etc.) within the department are:
- Uniquely identified (i.e. number and version)
- Written (e.g. in what format)
- Validated
- Approved
- Issued
- Reviewed (e.g. annually)

QUALITY CONTROL

Quality control is concerned with independent sampling and testing to confirm that a process meets stated requirements / specifications. This can take many forms including for example process and product control, individual worker assessment, equipment monitoring and reagent control. The information obtained should form the basis for statistical analysis, such as statistical process control, and be used for monitoring trends, performance and compliance. The information may also lead to actions being taken to bring a process back in control or be used as part of a continuous improvement programme. For example, in the National Blood Service the 'Guidelines for the Blood Transfusion Service in the UK' stipulates that 1% of blood component production should be subject to quality control and that a minimum of 75% of the results obtained should conform to the component's specifications.

STANDARD OPERATING PROCEDURES

A Standard Operating Procedure (SOP) is an instructional document, written to ensure a user can perform a task according to requirements. The author of the SOP should be familiar with both the procedure and the required format (in which the SOP should be written). All SOPs must be validated (i.e. the procedure is performed by a second party who follows the instructions as laid out in the document) to ensure the required outcome is achieved. In addition, the SOP must be approved by a responsible manager to ensure that the requirements of the department are being met in the document.

SOPs must be given a unique number, copies issued to named persons and be subject to regular review. It is also the responsibility of all persons to ensure that SOPs are followed correctly and are not subjected to unauthorised alterations.

PRE-ACCEPTANCE TESTING, VALIDATION AND CALIBRATION

All new items of equipment and purchased or in-house reagent batches must be subjected to a documented validation / acceptance process to demonstrate that they perform as expected, and to confirm that they are suitable for their intended use. It is also necessary to perform regular checks on critical items of equipment to ensure that their performance does not change with time. This is especially true of automated sampling equipment and temperature monitoring equipment, where these 'calibration' checks provide evidence that the equipment is continuing to meet specified requirements. A check failure would result in the item of equipment being removed from use until successful calibration was achieved.

MEDICINES AND HEALTHCARE PRODUCTS REGULATORY AGENCY (MHRA)

UK Blood Centres must be licensed under the Medicines Act and are inspected every two years (minimum) by the Medicines & Healthcare products Regulatory Agency (MHRA) who issue, and can revoke, their manufacturer's licence. The inspection is carried out using the European GMP Guide and the UK Guidelines for the Blood Transfusion Service (see Sources of Additional Information, for reference details), which identify the main criteria that have to be complied with. These points are usually incorporated into the Blood Centre's Quality Manual, which gives guidance to all departments.

CLINICAL PATHOLOGY ACCREDITATION UK Ltd (CPA) / HOSPITAL BLOOD BANKS AS THE 'KEEPER' OF BLOOD AND BLOOD PRODUCTS

Hospital Blood Banks and 'patient services' laboratories of Blood Centres can, if they wish, seek accreditation though the Clinical Pathology Accreditation (UK) Ltd (CPA) scheme. However, unlike the licensing of UK Blood Centres via the MHRA, the CPA process is not a mandatory process, but expected by the MHRA. The CPA inspection currently involves auditing against a series of standards, based on ISO 15189, identified in the CPA handbook, and this list should form the basis of a quality manual for each laboratory (or section), to enable them to meet these standards (see Sources of Additional Information, for reference details).

The CPA standards, based on a 'quality management' system, are as follows:

A   Organisation and quality management system
B   Personnel
C   Premises and Environment
D   Equipment, information systems and reagents
E   Pre-examination
F   Examination
G   Post examination
H   Evaluation and quality assurance

Under Product Liability law, each person or organisation in the chain of supply has a responsibility as a 'keeper' of a product, even if they are not the actual producers. Therefore, the hospital blood bank has a 'duty of care' to ensure that the blood and/or blood products that it keeps are suitable for their intended use. To do this the blood bank needs to maintain accurate records of what it receives and when (i.e. date and time), how these products are stored and how/when they are used, disposed, or returned to the supplier. The CPA standards cover these aspects and states that the hospital blood bank is responsible for the satellite refrigerators in operating theatres, delivery suits, etc., as well as the main blood bank. These must all be kept secure, that the blood should only be removed when it is needed and the person removing it must sign, together with the date and time, an appropriate register. It is necessary to retain records of blood cross-matched, etc., recorder charts from blood storage refrigerators and freezers used to store FFP and cryoprecipitate, for at least eleven years (see 'The retention and storage of pathological records and archives'; see Sources of Additional Information, for reference details). These charts should show the temperature of a simulated, or actual, pack of blood and/or blood product. Alarms should be activated by air temperature for blood storage refrigerators, but for frozen products, the sensor used for both the chart and alarm can be located on the surface of a product pack.

Other records

Records should be kept of the daily temperature of water baths, etc., quality control testing of cell washers, proficiency testing of staff and of the maintenance and calibration of centrifuges and other equipment carried out by service engineers. Reagent records are also required to show when a batch was received, how it was stored and if any material remained unused and was discarded. When in use, the reagent batch number should be included on the relevant work sheet.

SOME COMMON SENSE RULES

Each blood transfusion laboratory should have its own documented local policies for the selection and issue of blood and blood components, based on published guidelines. All staff must ensure that they are familiar with these policies. Relevant guidelines, standards and consensus statements are listed within the 'Sources of Additional Information'.

1. Be sure you have the correct Standard Operating Procedure (SOP) and that you follow it.
2. Be sure the correct materials (reagents, samples, etc.) are being used.
3. Be sure the correct equipment is used and that it is clean, operating correctly and calibrated.
4. Prevent contamination, mix-ups, and guard against labelling errors.
5. Work accurately and precisely, keeping the work area clean and uncluttered.
6. Be on the look out for (identified or suspected) mistakes, errors and bad practices and report any immediately ("covering-up" could cost lives!).
7. Keep clear and accurate records of each step; e.g. record the reaction results that you have obtained directly onto the worksheet.

Clear and accurate records enable everyone to:
- Be clear what they and others are doing.
- Confirm what has been done, and by whom.
- Investigate any complaints, defects, problems, etc.
- Help people take necessary corrective action.

GLOSSARY OF TERMS RELATING TO 'QUALITY'

There are a number of different definitions related to these subjects; those given below are from the International Quality Standard, the ISO 9000 series, or the International Council for Standardisation in Haematology (ICSH):

Quality
The totality of features and characteristics of a product or service that bear on its ability to satisfy stated or implied needs.

Quality Assurance
All those planned and systematic actions necessary to provide adequate confidence that a product or service will satisfy given requirements for quality.

Quality Control
The operational techniques and activities that are used to fulfil requirements for quality.

Quality Policy
The overall quality intentions and direction of an organisation as regards quality as formally expressed by top management.

Quality System
The organisational structure, responsibilities, processes and resources for implementing a quality policy.

Quality Audit
A systematic and independent examination to determine whether quality activities and related results comply with planned arrangements and whether these arrangements are implemented effectively and are suitable to achieve objectives.

Product Liability
A generic term used to describe the onus on a producer or others to make restitution for loss related to personal injury, property damage or other harm caused by a product or service (i.e. under the Consumer Protection Act).

Good Manufacturing Practice (GMP)
That part of quality assurance, which ensures that products are consistently produced and controlled to the quality standards appropriate to their intended use. (The GMP Guide, Rules and Guidance for Pharmaceutical Manufacturers, 1993, contains a section on the manufacture of blood products).

External Quality Assessment
This refers to a system of retrospectively and objectively comparing results obtained from different laboratories by means of exercises organised by an external agency (e.g. UK NEQAS).

Proficiency Testing
An essential part of good laboratory practice and internal quality control is to periodically test the proficiency of all workers by setting an exercise and comparing the results obtained from all participants with the expected results. Poor performance can then be recognised and identified.

Standard Operating Procedures (SOPs)
A series of written procedures (produced and issued as controlled documents) available for all activities performed in the blood transfusion laboratory. These documents should be linked into the in-service training programme of the department.

Finally:
Having read this training manual, done the exercises and answered the questions, you should have acquired a basic 'theoretical' understanding of how to perform the essential tasks in the Blood Transfusion laboratory. However, as with all things, there is no substitute for experience; practice makes perfect!

QUESTIONS - SECTION 15

1. Define the terms quality assurance and quality control.

2. What are the differences between internal and external quality schemes?

3. In what ways are the hospital blood banks "keepers" of blood and blood products?

4. What is CPA and what does it do?

5. What is the MHRA and what does it do?

6. Why are SOPs important? What are the possible consequences of not following a particular SOP?

7. Identify what documents control a 'Quality System'.

8. Identify the essential aspects of a Standard Operating Procedure (SOP) document.

9. Define Good Manufacturing Practice (GMP).

10. Why are clear and accurate records important?

SECTION 16

GLOSSARY OF TERMS

Adsorption

The process by which an antibody is removed from serum/plasma. That is, a serum/plasma rendered free of antibody is said to have been adsorbed. Red cells that have bound an antibody from a serum are said to have adsorbed that antibody. It is now common to use only the term adsorb and not distinguish between the terms adsorb and absorb.

Agglutination

The clumping together of red cells into visible aggregates (micro- and macroscopically) by antigen-antibody reactions.

AHG

An abbreviation for Anti-Human Globulin (Coomb's) reagent / test.

Albumin

In blood group serology, this term usually refers to 20% bovine albumin. Used to enhance certain antigen-antibody reactions, (in albumin displacement techniques) particularly those of the Rh system antibodies when present in a patient's serum/plasma together with other antibodies (i.e. a complex mixture)

Allele, Alleleomorph or Allelic gene

An alternative form of a series of genes that can occupy a single locus on either of a pair of homologous chromosomes. Normally the gene products (expressed in terms of red cell antigens) are antithetical.

Amorph

A gene that apparently has no function. Because it is seldom possible in immunohaematology, to differentiate between a gene that does not function and one that functions but whose product cannot be recognised in serological tests (i.e. no antibody to detect the product) the term silent allele is now preferred.

Antibody

A serum protein, produced as the result of the introduction of a foreign antigen, that has the ability to combine with (and in many cases lead to the destruction of) the cells carrying the antigen that stimulated its production. Blood group antibodies made by persons who have never been exposed to foreign red cells via transfusion, pregnancy or injection are made in response to the introduction of structurally similar antigens on substances other than red cells.

Antigen

A substance that when introduced into the circulation of a subject lacking the antigen, can stimulate the production of a specific antibody.

Autoantibody

An antibody that agglutinates or sensitises the red cells of the antibody donor, and may agglutinate or sensitise the red cells of other individuals.

Blood group substance
A non-red cell antigenic substance having the ability to neutralise a specific antibody, e.g. ABH substances in saliva.

Buffy coat
The thin layer of white cells and platelets which separates plasma from red cells when blood is centrifuged at high g-force.

Compatibility test ("Crossmatch")
A test carried out between serum/plasma and red cells to ensure they are non-reactive. Usually this term refers to the direct test between a patient's serum and the donor's red cells.

Complement
A series of alpha, beta and gamma globulins present in all normal sera. Some antibodies activate complement once they have complexed with antigen. Activation of the complement pathway serves as the effector mechanism by which cells coated with complement components are removed from the circulation by macrophages.

Complete Antibody
An antibody capable of causing agglutination in a saline medium. Usually IgM.

Cross-reacting antibody
An antibody that can combine with an antigen apparently different from the one that elicited its production, because the two antigens share structures that are similar in shape and charge.

Cytomegalovirus (CMV)
A human herpes-like virus, associated with white cells. Some blood donations are routinely screened for anti-CMV. Certain immunocompromised patients must receive CMV negative blood products.

Dominant gene
A gene that is expressed, in terms of antigenic production, when present in double or single dose.

Dosage effect
The difference in amount of antigen made when two like genes are present compared to the amount made when only one is present. Recognised by the reactions (in certain techniques) of some antibodies that are dependent on the amount of antigen present for the strength of their reaction.

Elution
A process, involving the destruction of the bonds between antigen and antibody, by which antibody molecules (previously adsorbed onto a red cell surface) are removed and are made available for further examination or use.

Epitope
The portion of the antigen with which the antibody molecules combine. A single antigen may contain many epitopes.

Extravascular haemolysis
The removal of intact red cells from the blood stream by the cells of the reticuloendothelial system; principally within the liver and spleen.

Gene
The basic unit of inheritance that determines the production or non-production of a character. It may be necessary that a series of genes be inherited in order that a recognisable character (such as a blood group antigen) is produced.

Genotype
A list of genes present. Very often a genotype represents interpretation of which genes are thought to be present, based on observed serological findings (phenotype).

Haemolysin
An antibody capable of destroying red cells in the presence of complement.

Haemolysis
The breaking down of the red cell with the liberation of the haemoglobin (see also intravascular haemolysis and extravascular haemolysis).

Haplotype
Genes, residing on one of the pair of homologous chromosomes, that usually travel together (gene complex).

Hemizygote
The presence of only one gene (of a possible pair) that influences the determination of a particular trait.

Heterozygote
An individual with dissimilar alleles at a given locus on homologous chromosomes.

Homozygote
An individual with identical alleles at a given locus on homologous chromosomes.

Immunoglobulin
Protein, or more specifically gamma globulin, of which antibodies are made. Major types involved in the production of blood group antibodies are IgG, IgM and IgA. Others, IgD and IgE, may be involved in the production of non-blood group antibodies.

Inhibition
The process of preventing an antibody from reacting by adding, to the serum containing the antibody, a substance capable of combining with, and hence neutralising, the antibody.

In vitro
Outside the body (in the transfusion laboratory test), meaning literally "in-glass".

In vivo
Within the body.

Incomplete antibody
An antibody that attaches to its specific antigen on the red cell surface but that is unable to cause agglutination in a saline medium. Usually IgG.

Intravascular haemolysis
The rupture of intact red cells in the blood stream by complement activation, resulting in the release of haemoglobin into the plasma.

Lectin
An extract usually made from seeds that has the ability to react with red cells. Lectins commonly used in blood group serology have specificity for known red cell antigens, e.g. *Dolichos biflorus* anti-A$_1$. Many others are known to agglutinate all red cells.

Linkage disequilibrium
A situation in which some haplotypes are more common than others because of unequal distribution of some alleles with others that are at closely linked loci or sub-loci.

Linked genes
Genes that travel together from parent to offspring. The degree of linkage is directly related to the closeness of loci to each other on the chromosome.

Leucodepletion
The process of removing white cells from blood donations / blood products by filtration, to a level below 5 million white cells per product.

Maximum Surgical Blood Order Schedule (MSBOS)
A schedule that determines the normal qualities of blood routinely issued for different surgical (medical) procedures by hospital transfusion laboratories.

Medicines & Healthcare products Regulatory Agency (MHRA)
UK body responsible for the licensing of pharmaceuticals and medicines production, which also therefore includes the UK Blood Services.

Monoclonal antibody
An antibody in which all molecules are identical since they have been produced by immunocytes belonging to a single clone. Monoclonal antibodies may be made (*in vivo*) in certain pathological conditions, but are now commonly produced in vitro using hybridomas. Each molecule complexes with the same portion (epitope) of the antigen.

National External Quality Assessment Scheme (NEQAS)
A scheme that provides standard control (test) samples to allow the independent monitoring of the performance of UK laboratories.

Non-specific
In transfusion science, this term is usually used to describe the joining of two substances (such as red cells and serum protein) in the absence of a specific reaction (such as an antibody-antigen reaction), e.g. random reaction of protein with cephalosporin treated red cells. A "non-specific antibody" is really an antibody of undetermined specificity, since when an antigen and antibody combine, the reaction always has specificity.

Peripheral Blood Stem Cells (PBSC)
An alternative to bone marrow donation, whereby haemopoietic progenitor cells (which give rise to all other blood cells) are mobilised from the marrow into the blood stream by treatment of the donor with a growth factor and collected by the use of apheresis methodology.

Phenotype
A list of antigens, shown by direct test observation to be present on an individual's red cells. Can be used to infer the probable genotype of the individual. Red cells can be phenotyped, they cannot be genotyped.

Polyagglutinable red cells
Red cells which are agglutinated by most normal adult human sera irrespective of the ABO groups involved (i.e. including group AB sera), but are rarely agglutinated by the serum of the individual from whom the red cells are obtained.

Polyclonal antibody
The type of antibody made in a normal *in vivo* alloimmune (and sometimes autoimmune) response. Made by many different clones of immunocytes so that it is a mixture of slightly different antibody molecules which vary in terms of binding constants, affinity and sometimes in terms of specificity since the different molecules may combine with different portions (epitopes) of the antigen.

Polymorphism
The existence in a population of more than one phenotype for any character or set of characters.

Prozone
A situation in which an antibody reacts more strongly when diluted than when used in the undiluted (raw) state.

Recessive gene
A gene whose presence is directly recognisable only in homozygotes.

Rouleaux
A property of some sera or certain compounds (e.g. dextrans), which causes red cells to stack together like piles of coins. It may be slight or gross, but in either condition may be mistaken for true agglutination.

Sensitised red cells
Red cells coated with but not agglutinated by an (IgG) antibody.

Specificity
The property of an antibody that enables it to combine with one but not other antigens. Specificity depends on the shape and goodness of fit relative to the antigen.

Thermal amplitude
The temperature range over which an antibody is active.

Titre
The greatest dilution of a serum/plasma, which still has sufficient antibody present to react with the corresponding antigen in a detectable manner. Titre is a measure of the strength of an antibody.

Variant Creutzfeldt-Jakob Disease (vCJD)
A fatal disease of the brain/central nervous system which is a variant of classical CJD and which is believed to have been derived in the UK from bovine spongiform encephalopathy (BSE) in cattle (i.e. 'mad cow' disease).

Washed red cells
Red cells freed of plasma or serum by repeated centrifuging through fresh volumes of phosphate buffered saline (PBS).

SOURCES OF ADDITIONAL INFORMATION

SELECTED WEBSITES

The American Association of Blood Banks publishes books and standards in the transfusion field:
http://www.aabb.org

The Association of Clinical Scientists is what you would expect and co-ordinates with HPC on registration of all kinds of Clinical Scientists:
http://www.assclinsci.org

The British Blood Transfusion Society:
http://www.bbts.org.uk

The British Committee for Standards in Haematology holds guidelines in this field – there is a transfusion section:
http://www.bcshguidelines.com

The Centre for Disease Control is a good source if statistics reports and guidance on all forms of infection, with a somewhat US bias. It also publishes the Morbidity and Mortality Weekly Report (http://www.cdc.gov/mmwr)
http://www.cdc.gov

The Chief Scientists Office in London provides updates on careers, research, etc.:
http://www.dh.gov.uk/AboutUs/HeadsOfProfession/ChiefScientificOfficer/fs/en

Clinical Pathology Accreditation undertakes inspection of diagnostic laboratories throughout the UK as well as elsewhere:
http://www.cpa-uk.co.uk

Food & Drug Administration are the US regulators:
http://www.fda.gov

The Health Professions Council deal with State Registration in the UK of Biomedical Scientists, Clinical Scientists, etc.:
http://www.hpc-uk.org

The Institute of Biomedical Science provide education and standards for biomedical Scientists
http://www.ibms.org

The International Blood Group Reference Laboratory site has a lot of good links to other websites of interest, books and educational materials:
http://www.bloodnet.nbs.nhs.uk/ibgrl/

The Network for Advancement of Transfusion Alternatives while sponsored by an erythropoietin manufacturer provides up to date reviews, meetings and links on alternatives to standard transfusion:
http://www.nataonline.com

The National (English) Blood Service Website includes updates, hospital guidelines, etc.:
http://www.bloodnet.nbs.nhs.uk

PubMed (based at the National Library of Medicine in Washington) is the most used site when searching for individual papers – just type in name subject, year or combinations at the top and hit search:
http://www.ncbi.nlm.nih.gov/entrez/query.fcgi?CMD=search&DB=PubMed

The Serious Hazards of Transfusion site contains the "SHOT" annual reports:
http://www.shotuk.org

The Scottish Intercollegiate Guidelines Network contains a number of guidelines of interest (e.g. on peri-operative transfusion):
http://www.sign.ac.uk

The UK Transfusion Guidelines site contains the "Red Book", the Handbook of Transfusion Medicine, as well as a number of other documents and links:
http://www.transfusionguidelines.org.uk

A SHORT LIST OF BOOKS ON TRANSFUSION SCIENCE

a. ABC of Transfusion
   Contreras M. (Ed.)
   BMJ Publishing Group. 3rd Edition. 1998   ISBN 0-7279-1209-7

b. AABB : Technical Manual
   American Association of Blood Banks
   AABB. 16th Edition. 2008.   ISBN 978-1-56395-260-9

c. Mollison's Blood Transfusion in Clinical Medicine
   Klein H. and Anstee D.
   Blackwell Scientific. 11th Edition. 2005.   ISBN: 0-6320-6454-4

d. Applied Blood Group Serology
   Issitt P.D. and Anstee D.J.
   Montgomery Scientific. 4th Edition. 1998.   ISBN 0-935643-05-2

e. Handbook of Transfusion Medicine
   McClelland D.B.L. (Ed.).
   The Stationery Office. 4th Edition. 2007.   ISBN 0-11-322677-2
   See *http://www.transfusionguidelines.org.uk*

f. Practical Transfusion Medicine
   Ed: Murphy M.F. and Pamphilon D.H.
   Blackwell. 2005   2nd Edition   ISBN: 1-40511844-X

g. Human Blood Groups
   Daniels G.
   Blackwell Scientific. 2nd Edition 2002   ISBN 0-6320-5646-0

h. Modern Transfusion Medicine
   Pamphilon D.H.
   CRC Press. 1995.   ISBN 0-8493-8922-4

i. Handbook of Blood Transfusion Therapy
Napier J.A.F
Wiley. 2nd Edition. 1995   ISBN 0-471-95378-4

j. Alloimmune Disorders of Pregnancy: Anaemia, Thrombocytopenia and Neutropenia
in the Fetus and Newborn
Hadley A.G. and Soothill A.G.
Cambridge University Press   ISBN 0-521-78120-5

k. Introduction to Blood Transfusion Technology
Armstrong B., Hardwick J., Raman L., Smart E. and Wilkinson R.
ISBT Science Series, Vol 3, No 2. June 2008   ISSN 0042-9007

l. Essential Guide to Blood Groups
Daniels G. and Bromilow I.
Blackwell Publishing. 2007   ISBN 978-1-4051-5349-2

m. Transfusion Microbiology
Ed: Barbara J.A.J., Regan F.A.M. and Contreras M.C.
Cambridge University Press. 2008.   ISBN 978-0-521-45393-6

n. Blood Group Antigens and Antibodies
Reid M.E. and Lomas-Francis C.
SBB Books. 2007.   ISBN-13 978-1-59572-103-7

The above list is by no means exhaustive, but is intended to give information regarding broad based textbooks on Transfusion Science, related to both specific as well as general topic areas.

ADDITIONAL INFORMATION SOURCES: RELEVANT GUIDELINES
(in published date order)
The BCSH website provides an up to date list and makes these guidelines available in their latest form: http://www.bcshguidelines.com

1. Guidelines for autologous transfusion
Clin Lab Haemat. 1988. 10, 193-201.

2. Guidelines for transfusion for massive blood loss
Clin Lab Haemat. 1988. 10, 265-273.

3. Guidelines on hospital blood bank documentation and procedures
BCSH.
Clin Lab Haemat. 1990. 12, 209-220 (Revised).

4. Guidelines for implementation of a Maximum Surgical Blood Order Schedule
Clin Lab Haemat. 1990. 12, 321-327.

5. Guidelines on product liability for the hospital blood bank
Clin Lab Haemat. 1990. 12, 329-344.

6. Guidelines for microplate techniques in liquid-phase blood grouping and antibody screening
Clin Lab Haemat. 1990. 12, 437-460.

7. Guidelines for autologous transfusion. 1. Pre-operative autologous donation
   BCSH.
   Transfusion Medicine. 1993. 3, 307-316

8. Recommendations for evaluation, validation and implementation of new techniques for blood grouping, antibody screening and cross-matching
   BCSH.
   Transfusion Medicine. 1995. 5, 145-150.

9. Guidelines on the investigation and management of thrombocytopenia in pregnancy and neonatal alloimmune thrombocytopenia
   British Journal of Haematology. 1996. 95, 21-26.

10. Guidelines for blood grouping and red cell antibody testing during pregnancy
    BCSH/BBTS.
    Transfusion Medicine. 1996. 6, 71-74.
    NOTE: See also addendum: Transfusion Medicine. 1999. 9, 99.

11. Guidelines on gamma irradiation of blood components for the prevention of Transfusion-Associated Graft-versus-Host Disease
    BCSH.
    Transfusion Medicine. 1996. 6, 261-271.

12. Guidelines on the clinical use of leucocyte-depleted blood components
    BCSH.
    Transfusion Medicine. 1998. 8, 59-71

13. The estimation of fetomaternal haemorrhage
    BCSH / Blood Transfusion Task Force / Haematology Task Force
    Transfusion Medicine. 1999. 9, 87-92

14. Recommendations for the use of anti-D immunoglobulin for Rh prophylaxis
    BCSH / Royal College of Obstetricians and Gynaecologists.
    Transfusion Medicine. 1999. 9, 93-97

15. The administration of blood and blood components and the management of transfused patients
    BCSH / Royal College of Nursing / Royal College of Surgeons of England.
    Transfusion Medicine. 1999. 9, 227-238

16. Guidelines for blood bank computing
    BCSH / Blood Transfusion Task Force
    Transfusion Medicine, 2000. 10, 307-314

17. Guidelines for the clinical use of red cell transfusions
    BCSH / Blood Transfusion Task Force
    British Journal of Haematology, 2001. 113, 24-31

18. Guidelines for the use of platelet transfusions
    BCSH
    British Journal of Haematology, 2003. 112, 10-23

19. Guidelines for compatibility procedures in blood transfusion laboratories
    BCSH / Blood Transfusion Task Force
    Transfusion Medicine, 2004. 14, 59-73

20. Transfusion guidelines for neonates and older children
Boulton F.
British Journal of Haematology, 2004. 114, 433-453
See also amendments to this Guideline:
http://hospital.blood.co.uk/library/pdf/amendments_*dec05.pdf*

21. Guidelines for the use of fresh-frozen plasma, cryoprecipitate and cryosupernatant
BCSH.
British Journal of Haematology, 2004. 126, 11-28
See also amendments to this Guideline:
http://hospital.blood.co.uk/library/pdf/amendments_*dec05.pdf*

ADDITIONAL INFORMATION SOURCES: CONSENSUS STATEMENTS

a. Leucocyte depletion of blood and blood components
Consensus Conference
Held at the Royal College of Physicians of Edinburgh, 18-19th March 1993.

b. Consensus statement on red cell transfusion
Transfusion Medicine. 1994. 4, 177-178
Royal College of Physicians.

c. Consensus statement on autologous transfusion
Transfusion Medicine. 1996. 6, 69-70.
Royal College of Physicians.

d. Consensus statement on anti-D prophylaxis
Transfusion Medicine. 1997. 7, 143-144
Royal College of Physicians / Royal College of Obstetricians and Gynaecologists.

e. Consensus conference on platelet transfusion
Royal College of Physicians of Edinburgh. 1997.

ADDITIONAL REFERENCES - VARIOUS

a. Guidelines for the Blood Transfusion Services in the United Kingdom
The Stationery Officer. 7th Edition. 2005. ISBN 0-1170-3371-5
See also http://www.transfusionguidelines.org.uk

b. Clinical Pathology Accreditation
Accreditation Handbook 2nd Edition. 2004. *(available on http://www.cpa-uk.co.uk)*
CPA (UK) Ltd. Sheffield.

c. The retention and storage of pathological records and archives
Royal College of Pathologists. 2nd Edition. 1999.

d. Serious Hazards of Transfusion - annual report
By: The Serious Hazards of Transfusion Steering Committee
SHOT Office, Plymouth Grove, Manchester M13 9LL
See also http://www.shot.org

e. Rules and Guidance for Pharmaceutical Manufacturers and Distributors 2002 (the "Orange Guide")
Medicines Control Agency. ISBN 0-1132-2559-8
This publication brings together the main pharmaceutical Regulations, Directives and guidance, including GMP and GDP, which manufacturers and wholesalers are expected to follow when making and distributing medicinal products in the European Union and European Economic Area.

f. ICH harmonised tripartite guideline for good clinical practice
Publication Date: 31st May 2005. ISBN: 1904255086

g. Statutory instrument 2005 No. 50. The Blood Safety and Quality Regulations (2005) (http://www.opsi.gov.uk/si/si2005/20050050.htm)
The Blood Safety and Quality Regulation (No 50) 2005, made under Section 2(2) of the European Communities Act 1972, transpose two European Union directives (2002/98/EC and 2004/33/EC) into UK law. The Blood Safety and Quality Regulations came into force from 8 November 2005.

h. Guidance note on the Blood Safety and Quality Regulation (No.50) 2005:
http://www.dh.gov.uk/assetRoot/04/11/80/09/04118009.pdf

i. The impact of the blood safety and quality regulation 2005 on hospital transfusion laboratories. The NHS operational impact group (OIG) report:
http://www.transfusionguidelines.org.uk/docs/pdfs/oig_report.pdf

ANSWERS

1. **List the major characteristics of IgG and IgM antibodies.**

	IgG	IgM
Molecular weight (approximate)	160,000	900,000
Placental transfer	Yes	No
Complement activation	Yes	Yes
Normal reaction temperature	37°C	4°C - 20°C
Primary response	Rare	Yes
Secondary response	Yes	Rare

2. **List the main factors affecting the uptake of antibody onto red cells (i.e. sensitisation of red cells).**
   Factors affecting the Primary Stage:
   a. Red cell (antigen) – Serum/plasma (antibody) ratio
   b. Ionic strength
   c. Temperature

3. **List the main factors affecting the agglutination of red cells.**
   Factors affecting the Secondary Stage:
   a. Gravity / Centrifugation
   b. Addition of aggregating agents, e.g. 20% bovine albumin or polybrene
   c. Use of Enzymes

4. **What is an anamnestic response?**
   This is an immune response produced by 'primed' (memory) B cells due to the exposure of a second dose of the same antigen, i.e. following a primary response. There appears to be a need for a time delay between the two antigenic exposures for the secondary response to be produced. The secondary response is independent of T cell involvement. This generally produces larger amounts of invariably IgG antibody, with little time delay, an antibody with improved affinity for the antigen, which has an increased reactivity (avidity) with its antigen.

5. **Why are IgG antibodies unable to agglutinate red cells in a saline medium?**
   The balance of the attractive forces of gravity and surface tension, balanced by the repulsive forces due to the net negative charges of red cells dictates a minimum distance between red cells in a saline medium. This repulsive force is such that the red cells cannot approach close enough to allow an IgG molecule to span the gap between them. An IgM antibody molecule is however large enough to span this gap and therefore IgM molecules are capable of causing agglutination of red cells in a saline medium, whereas (usually) IgG cannot.

6. **Why should homozygous red cells be used for antibody detection?**
   Generally, experiments have demonstrated that more antigen sites are present on red cells of the homozygote rather than the heterozygote phenotype. Therefore more antibodies are able to bind to the homozygous phenotype cell, which will increase the sensitivity of the antigen-antibody reaction.

7. **Which red cell antigens are glycoprotein and which are carbohydrate?**
   Carbohydrate: ABO, Lewis, P_1, H and I
   Protein: MNS, Rh, Lutheran, Kell, Duffy and Kidd

8. **How are 'naturally occurring' antibodies produced?**
   Via the presence of antigenic material (similar to red cell antigens) on the surface of bacteria or viruses, or present in food. As a result, apparent red cell antibodies may be stimulated to be produced without the infusion of human red cells. This process accounts for the production of ABO antibodies and occasionally the antibodies of other blood group antigens.

9. **Define the terms 'antigen' and 'antibody'.**
   Antigen: Any substance, which in appropriate biological circumstances, can stimulate the formation of an antibody.
   Antibody: Proteins (immunoglobulins) occurring in body fluids which are produced in response to the introduction of foreign antigen.

10. **What is the factor that defines whether an antibody reacts best at 4°C-20°C or 37°C?**
    The nature of the bonds which bind the antigen and antibody together. If these are exothermic (give off heat during their formation), such as hydrogen bonds, then they work better at colder temperatures since the heat is dissipated from the site of the reaction quickly.

SECTION 2

1. **Explain intravascular red cell removal.**
   Intravascular removal involves haemolysis (rupture) of the red cells in the blood stream by complement activation, releasing Hb into the plasma.

2. **Explain extravascular red cell removal.**
   Extravascular removal involves removal of IgG and/or complement (C3) coated red cells from the circulation by macrophages of the reticuloendothelial system within the liver and spleen.

3. **How are red cells removed by macrophages in the liver and spleen?**
   Tissue bound macrophages have membrane receptors for IgG and the complement component C3. If either or both of these molecules are bound to the surface of a red cell, then the red cell becomes bound to the macrophage. This results in either the red cell being removed from the circulation or part of the red cell membrane is removed and the spherocytic red cell released into the circulation. Macrophages with C3 receptors are principally located in the liver; those with IgG receptor are principally in the spleen.

4. **What activates the classic complement pathway?**
   The binding of either a single IgM antibody molecule or two IgG antibody molecules very close together on the red cell membrane. Once bound, the Fc portion of the antibody activates and binds C1, the first component of the complement cascade. Not all antibodies are however capable of causing complement activation (Rh does not).

5. **Why is complement not able to be activated *in vitro* using anticoagulated (plasma) samples?**
   The complement component C1 requires calcium ions to maintain its structure. EDTA/citrate binds calcium and therefore in the presence of these anticoagulants C1 is inactive, means that C1 cannot be bound and the complement classic pathway cannot be activated.

6. **Identify the three phases of the Classic complement pathway**
   The 'activation', the 'amplification' and the 'membrane attack' phases.

7. **How many IgG or IgM antibody molecules are required to activate C1?**
   C1 is activated by one IgM molecule binding with its antigen, or two IgG molecules binding close together on the red cell membrane.

8. **What clinical effects define an antibody as 'clinically significant'?**
   The fact that it is capable of producing either a (haemolytic) transfusion reaction and/or HDFN.

9. **How do 'clinically significant' antibodies react *in vitro*?**
   Identified classically as reacting at 37°C by IAT.

10. **How is complement inactivated?**
    Complement can be inactivated by the presence of anticoagulants (affects C1), heat (affects C1 and C2) and relatively long periods of storage *in vitro*. *In vivo* it can be inactivated by the presence of inactivator proteins (e.g. C1 INH) and the short half-life of some of the activated complement proteins.

SECTION 3

1. **Tabulate the expected reactions of the four ABO blood groups with anti-A, anti-B, anti-A,B together with A_1, A_2, B and O red cells.**

GROUP	ANTISERA			RED CELLS			
	Anti-A	Anti-B	Anti-A,B	A_1	A_2	B	O
A	4	0	4	0	0	4	0
B	0	4	4	4	4	0	0
AB	4	4	4	0	0	0	0
O	0	0	0	4	4	4	0

2. **Tabulate the controls you would use for routine ABO grouping and their expected reactions.**

ANTISERA		RED CELLS		
	A$_1$	[A$_2$ optional]	B	O
Anti-A	4	[4]	0	0
Anti-B	0	[0]	4	0
[Anti-A,B optional]	[4]	[4]	[4]	[0]
[Reagent control optional]	[0]	[0]	[0]	[0]

3. **What are the possible ABO genotypes of the offspring from the following matings?**
   a. Group B x group AB   :   AO BB AB BO
   b. Group B x group A$_2$:   A$_2$O A$_2$B OO BO
   c. Group B x group A$_1$:   A$_1$B A$_2$B OO BO A$_1$O A$_2$O
   (answers do not include the A$_3$ and A$_x$ subgroups of A)

4. **What possible genotypes produce the A$_1$ A$_2$ A$_3$ and A$_x$ phenotypes?**

Phenotype	Possible genotypes				
A$_1$	A_1A_1	A_1O	A_1A_2	A_1A_3	A_1A_x
A$_2$	A_2A_2	A_2O	A_2A_3	$A_2 A_x$	
A$_3$	A_3A_3	A_3O			
A$_x$	A_xA_x	A_xO			

5. **Which ABO blood group has the most H substance and which has the least?**
   Group O have the most since none is converted to A or B antigens. Group A$_1$ and A$_1$B have the least and as such it is these groups who occasionally produce a non-clinically significant cold reacting anti-H.

6. **Anti-A$_1$ can be produced by which of the A subgroups?**
   All subgroups of A with the exception of A$_1$ (e.g. A$_2$ A$_3$ A$_x$) are able to produce this antibody. Approximately 2% of group A$_2$ (and approximately 25% of group A$_2$B) produce anti-A$_1$. Group A$_x$ frequently produces it.

7. **Why is the ABO blood group system the most clinically important?**
   Due to the universal presence in adults of ABO antibodies, i.e. 97% of the population (all but group AB) have an antibody, whilst approximately 55% of the population have either or both A and B antigens, increasing the chance of the transfusion of A or B incompatible red cells should an error occur. The antibodies are clinically significant, capable of readily activating complement and causing intravascular red cell destruction.

8. **Tabulate the expected reactions of a group O and group O$_h$.**

Grp	Routine ABO grouping							Non-routine
	Anti-A	Anti-B	Anti-A,B	Auto	A RBCs	B RBCs	O RBCs	Anti-H
O	0	0	0	0	4	4	0	4
O$_h$	0	0	0	0	4	4	4*	0

   * = due to the presence of clinically significant anti-H

9. **What are the approximate frequencies of each of the four ABO blood groups in the UK?**
   A = 43%   B = 9%   O = 45%   AB = 3%

10. **What chemical structures comprise the ABO antigens?**
    Carbohydrates (sugars) - linked to lipids on the red cell (i.e. as glycolipid) and protein in the serum as glycoprotein. The H structure is fucose linked to a terminal galactose, the A and B structures are terminally linked N-acetyl-D-galactosamine and D-galactose respectively.

ABO phenotype / genotype interpretation

No	Phen	Reason	Genotype options
1	O	No RBC antigen reactions / anti-A,B in serum	OO
2	A$_1$	RBC reactions vs. anti-A; -A,B; -A$_1$ / anti-B in serum	$A^1A^1 / A^1A^2 / A^1O$ **
3	A$_1$B	RBC reactions vs. anti-A; -A,B; -B; -A$_1$ / no antibodies in serum	A^1B
4	B	RBC reactions vs. anti-B; -A,B / anti-A in serum	BB / BO
5	A$_2$	RBC reactions vs. anti-A; -A,B (but not anti-A$_1$) / anti-B and an antibody reacting against A$_2$ RBCs in serum (possible anti-A$_1$)	A^2A^2 / A^2O *
6	O	No RBC antigen reactions / anti-A,B in serum + a positive reaction vs. group O RBCs (RT reactive antibody ? specificity)	OO

193

7	A$_2$B	RBC reactions vs. anti-A; -A,B; -B (but not anti-A$_1$) / no antibodies in serum	A^2B ∧∧
8	B	RBC reactions vs. anti-B; -A,B / No anti-A in serum, possibly due to the age of the patient or another reason	BB / BO
9	A$_2$	RBC reactions vs. anti-A; -A,B (but not anti-A$_1$) / anti-B in serum	A^2A^2 / A^2O *
10	A$_2$B	RBC reactions vs. anti-A; -A,B; -B (but not anti-A$_1$) / an antibody reacting against A$_2$ RBCs in serum (possible anti-A$_1$)	A^2B ∧∧

* These results could also indicate a rarer sub-group of A than group A$_2$, for example groups A$_3$ or A$_x$ since the reactions with these monoclonal grouping antisera may well be the same.

** Does not include other genotype options including A^3 or A^x

∧∧ May be a different weak A subtype and not necessarily A$_2$

SECTION 4

1. **What percentage of the UK population is D positive and D negative?**
Approximately 85% are D positive and 15% are D negative.

2. **Why is it not necessary to test patient samples for weak D (D^u) antigen?**
It is less important to detect weak D types in recipients, since the consequences of grouping a recipient as D negative will result in that person, who is actually D positive, receiving D negative blood. Individuals who have weak D antigen expression are incapable of forming anti-D.

3. **State which CcDEe antigens are represented by the following haplotypes:**
   a. R$_1$ CDe
   b. R$_2$ cDE
   c. r   cde
   d. r′   Cde
   e. r′′   cdE
   f. R$_o$ cDe

4. **Why is the D antigen believed to be so strongly immunogenic?**
Due to the fact that D negative people have no D product i.e. completely lack the D protein - this is unlike other blood group system antigens which normally vary by only a small number of amino-acids within a protein which is otherwise the same.

5. **Can 'weak D' and 'variant D' types produce anti-D?**
Weak D type people are D positive and (classically) are not capable of producing anti-D (i.e. they produce normal D antigens but in smaller quantities than normal).
Variant D types produce abnormal D antigens that lack parts of the normal D antigenic structure. As such, some of these with little antigenic expression (e.g. category VI types) are capable of producing anti-D, an antibody against the parts of the D antigen that they lack, which is capable of reacting with normal D antigens.

6. **What approximate percentage of the UK population are O Rh D negative, O Rh D positive, A Rh D negative and A Rh D positive?**
O Rh D neg: 6.75%
O Rh D pos: 38.25%
A Rh D neg: 6.5%
A Rh D pos: 36.6%

7. **Which of the Rh antibodies are capable of causing red cell destruction of incompatible red cells?**
All are capable of doing so if reactive in AHG (c.f. enzyme only reactive) - extravascular removal.

8. **What genotype are the fetal D positive red cells, which stimulate a D negative woman to produce anti-D?**
The mother must be D negative (*dd*), therefore all D positive babies of D negative mothers must have received their *D* gene from the father and a *d* gene from their mother and must therefore be heterozygote *Dd*.

9. **What are the phenotype and most likely genotypes from the following Rh grouping results?**

	Anti- D C c E e	Phenotype	Most probable genotype
Sample A	+ + + + +	CcDEe	CDe/cDE (R_1R_2)
Sample B	- - + + +	cdEe	cdE/cde ($r''r$)
Sample C	+ + - - +	CDe	CDe/CDe (R_1R_1)
Sample D	+ - + + +	cDEe	cDE/cde (R_2r)
Sample E	- + + - +	Ccde	Cde/cde ($r'r$)

10. **Which are the Rh antibodies most likely cause HDFN?**
Anti-D (as anti-D, anti-C+D, anti-D+E or anti-C+D+E) and anti-c

ABO / RhD groups - interpretation

No	Group	Comments
1	A neg	-
2	B pos	-
3	O pos	Weak positive reactions with the two anti-D sera (not significant – transfused D+ RBCs). Note: if reactions are so weak as to be undecided, transfuse D negative RBCs in an emergency and refer to a reference laboratory.
4	A neg	Positive reaction with group A_1 red cells (? presence of anti-A_1).
5	O neg	Positive reactions with O red cells indicates presence of an unknown antibody specificity reactive at RT.
6	AB pos	-
7	A pos	Mixed field result indicates the possible presence of some O+ red cells in an A+ patient (? post-transfusion) – transfused cells are D+ and not D negative since there is no mixed field reactions with anti-D sera / transfused cells are group O and patient is group A since anti-B present in serum/plasma. Alternative explanation is that the patient is a weak subtype of A (unlikely since anti-A and anti-A,B used are monoclonal).
8	B ?	Possibly variant D type (if two D grouping tests involve anti-D sera from different clones). Requires further investigation since true group unknown – refer to a reference laboratory. If an emergency transfuse group D negative RBCs.
9	AB neg	Positive results with group A_1 RBC reactions (? presence of anti-A_1).
10	A pos	Positive reactions with A_2 and O RBCs - antibody specificity unknown, possibly anti-H based on variable strength of results with these cells.
11	B neg	Weak anti-A reactions (not significant).
12	O neg	No anti-A,B (?cause – age, i.e. a baby)

SECTION 5

1. **What is an autologous control and what is its purpose?**
This control is the patient's red cells reacted against the patient's serum, by the same technique as the test. This control should be negative, since a person cannot normally produce an antibody to the corresponding antigen present on their red cells. It is used to detect the presence of an autoantibody specificity.

2. **What is a reagent control and what is its purpose?**
This is used when antigen grouping a red cell sample with a known specificity antiserum. If monoclonal reagents are used, the manufacturer's "Reagent Control" must be used as a control, whereas, if a human polyclonal reagent is used, AB serum, which has been previously tested and found to contain no antibodies to any blood group antigen, is chosen for this control. The reagent control or AB serum is reacted against the test red cell sample by the same technique used for the grouping sera. If this control is positive, the test results cannot be relied upon. The reagent control is used to identify red cells, which are capable of reacting "non-specifically", e.g. polyagglutinable.

3. **What controls should be used when performing an enzyme technique?**
Positive: Weak anti-D with D positive enzyme treated red cells.
Negative: AB serum with D positive enzyme treated red cells.

4. **Describe the controls required for ABO grouping.**
The antisera used for the cell group, i.e. anti-A and anti-B (and -A,B if used) should be reacted against the red cell samples used for the serum group, i.e. A_1 and B (and O) in a checkerboard manner, using the same technique criteria as the test. The expected results must be obtained, i.e.

	A₁	B	O
Anti-A	4	0	0
Anti-B	0	4	0
Anti-A,B	4	4	0

5. **Identify the controls required for Rh D grouping.**

   The two anti-D sera used for D grouping should be reacted with D positive (R₁r) red cell sample and a D negative (rr) red cell sample, using the same technique criteria as the test. The expected results must be obtained.

6. **Identify the controls required for Duffy grouping a patient's red cell sample using anti-Fyᵃ reagent by an AHG technique.**

   Positive and negative grouping reagent control red cell samples should be used; the positive being preferably the heterozygote Fy(a+b+) and the negative being Fy(a-b+). These should be set up and tested using the same technique criteria as the test. In addition, IgG sensitised red cells should be used to validate negative test (and control) results if a tube IAT is used.

7. **What does a positive reaction of a patient's red cell sample with antibody-free AB serum indicate?**

   That the patient's red cells are capable of reacting with any serum sample, irrespective of the presence of specific antibody (i.e. are polyagglutinable). Any results obtained with these red cells against specific antisera are therefore unreliable.

8. **What are the two stages of a 'two stage' enzyme technique and what do they achieve?**

   The first stage involves an initial enzyme pre-modification of the red cell sample(s). The enzyme treatment is then stopped, excess enzyme removed and the red cell sample standardised. This stage removes protein from the red cell surface, which reduces the negative charge, allowing the red cells to get closer together, within the span of an IgG molecule.

   The second stage is the enzyme treated red cells added to the patient's serum/plasma in a direct agglutination technique –. If the serum/plasma contains an IgG alloantibody, then they will cause the agglutination of the cells. The reactivity of some protein antigens is enhanced by the enzyme treatment (e.g. Rh) whilst others are reduced or removed altogether (e.g. Duffy).

9. **Why are equal volumes of serum/plasma and red cells used in a LISS technique?**

   The final (working) ionic strength of LISS is based on the fact that the red cells suspended in the LISS as a 1.5% - 2% solution will be added to an equal volume of serum/plasma. An increased volume of serum/plasma will alter this final ionic strength. As a consequence it is important that equal volumes are maintained.

10. **What methods can be employed to increase the sensitivity of the direct agglutination technique in normal saline?**

    The antigen – antibody reaction sensitivity can be increased by increasing the ratio of antibody to antigen (using more serum/plasma), allowing more antibody per red cell to bind. Increasing the incubation time and/or use of centrifugation.

SECTION 6

1. **Indicate and explain the main steps in an indirect (tube) antiglobulin test.**

   TECHNIQUE STAGES | EXPLANATION
   - In a 75 x 12mm glass tube place :
     2 drops of serum/plasma }
     2 drops of red cells in LISS } Maintains equal volumes
   - Mix the contents well. }
   - Incubate at 37°C for 15-20 minutes. } Antigen - antibody reaction
   - Look for haemolysis and/or agglutination.   Identify direct reaction
   - Wash the red cells 4 times in saline.   Remove excess Ig
   - Add 2 drops of AHG reagent, mix.   Binds with RBC bound Ig
   - Gently centrifuge the tube.   Increase speed of reaction
   - Read and record the reactions.
   - To negative tests add one drop of IgG sensitised red cells, mix and gently centrifuge then read.
   - Agglutination should now be present. If negative, the test must be repeated. This identifies false negative reactions (no free AHG reagent).

2. **List five reasons why a false positive result may be obtained in an IAT.**
   - Presence of particulate matter, dust, plastic particles, etc., in the tube.
   - Presence of substances in the saline that leads to non-specific agglutination of the red cells (e.g. colloidal silica or metal ions).
   - Poorly absorbed polyclonal AHG reagent, which will react with un-coated human red cells.
   - Cross-contamination from one tube to another, or from poorly cleaned cell washers.
   - Red cells with a positive direct antiglobulin test.
   - Over-centrifugation.
   - Failure to detect agglutination before washing the cells.
   - Wrong / incorrect LISS concentration (i.e. too low).

3. **List five reasons why a false negative result may be obtained in an IAT.**
   - Inadequate washing of the red cells, i.e. as little as a 1 in 4,000 dilution of serum/plasma in saline is capable of neutralising an equivalent volume of AHG reagent.
   - Failure to add AHG reagent.
   - Inactive AHG reagent due to inadequate storage conditions, contamination with bacteria or serum, use after the reagent's expiry date, etc.
   - Loss of antigens from the red cell surface due to prolonged or inadequate sample/red cell storage.
   - Inactive serum/plasma due to inadequate storage conditions, e.g. repeated freezing and thawing, etc.
   - Inadequate incubation time or temperature.
   - Presence of fibrin clots; these will exude serum even after washing and will neutralise the AHG reagent.
   - Cross-contamination with other tubes (e.g. as when the tube is inverted against the finger, which is contaminated with serum or blood).
   - Un-buffered saline at too low a pH (antibodies elute from red cells at a low pH).
   - Excess antigen, i.e. too many red cells in the reaction mixture.
   - Leaving the cells too long before adding the AHG reagent (weakly bound antibodies may elute from the red cells) or after adding the AHG reagent (positive IATs, due to IgG coating, becoming weaker on standing).
   - Wrong / incorrect LISS concentration (i.e. too high).

4. **How do IgG sensitised red cells work in controlling the AHG test?**
   They act to control negative AHG test results in identifying that they are true negatives and not false negatives. In a true negative, there is free unused AHG reagent left which is capable of reacting with the IgG sensitised red cells when added. The most common cause of a false negative result is that the AHG reagent has been neutralised by free immunoglobulin remaining in the test as a result of poor washing. In such a situation, there is no free unused AHG reagent available to agglutinate the IgG coated red cells when added.

5. **What is the difference between an IAT and DAT?**
   The IAT involves the pre-incubation of serum/plasma and red cell sample prior to washing and AHG reagent addition, which therefore detects *in vitro* reaction of antibody with antigen, e.g. in a crossmatch. The DAT does not involve any incubation of serum/plasma and red cells as it is designed to detect an *in vivo* reaction of antibody and antigen, e.g. on fetal red cells to detect possible HDFN.

6. **What is the advantage of using a 'broad spectrum' AHG reagent?**
   'Broad spectrum' AHG reagent, as well as containing anti-IgG also contains anti-C3. This is present so as to enhance the detection of any antigen-antibody reaction, which also causes the binding of complement components, since the two types of antibody will be able to cross-link the sensitised red cells.

7. **What is the primary difference in the use of serum or plasma samples for the AHG test?**
   Serum allows complement activation by an antigen-antibody reaction to occur (if it is capable to do so) whereas plasma does not since it inhibits C1. As such, if plasma is used, only IgG is able to be detected on the red cells and 'broad spectrum' AHG serum is of no additional benefit.

8. **If no red cells are detected on the surface, within or at the bottom of an AHG gel test used for a crossmatch, what does this signify and why?**
   Assuming that the red cells were added in the first place (this should be checked at the time) then it indicates that the red cells have haemolysed. This could have occurred as a result of an ABO incompatible crossmatch (e.g. group O patient and group A donor red cells). As such, this situation must be taken as a positive result and the groups / clerical aspects of the crossmatch re-checked and the test repeated.

9. **What should be added to each tube position of a cell washer to control its action?**
One drop of IgG coated red cells and one drop of AB serum. If the cell washer is working correctly then the AB serum will be washed away, leaving no free immunoglobulin. The added AHG reagent will then result in a positive result. Any tube not giving this will result in the cell washer being taken out of service, cleaned, fresh saline placed in the reservoir and the quality control tests repeated.

10. **What concentration of serum is capable of inhibiting AHG reagent added to an AHG test resulting in a false-negative result?**
A 1 in 4,000 dilution is capable of neutralising an equivalent volume of AHG reagent.

SECTION 7

1. **Explain the difference between an 'alloantibody' and an 'autoantibody'.**
An alloantibody may be produced as a result of a normal immune response to a foreign red cell antigen, following an immunising event such as a transfusion or pregnancy. An autoantibody is produced as a result of a rare abnormal event, directed against the person's own red cells, which can lead to auto-immune haemolytic anaemia (AIHA). In addition, some patients produce autoantibodies as a result of taking certain drugs, resulting in drug associated (or drug induced) haemolytic anaemia.

2. **List the most commonly identified IgG antibody specificities to be found in patient's serum/plasma.**

Antibody Specificity	Approx. % patients positive
ANTI-D	0.3%
ANTI-C+D	0.2%
ANTI-D+E	0.06%
ANTI-E	0.5%
ANTI-c	0.1%
ANTI-K	0.4%
ANTI-Fy^a	0.04%
ANTI-Jk^a	0.02%
ANTI-S	0.01%

3. **Why is homozygosity of antigenic expression, for certain antigens, important for antibody screening cells?**
For transfusion recipients, a positive antibody screening test indicates a risk of a transfusion reaction, irrespective of the compatibility test result, since the red cells used for antibody detection may be able to detect the patient's antibody better than the donor's red cells due to antigen dosage effects. Dosage effect occurs due to the production of more antigen by the homozygote genotype than the heterozygote genotype, e.g. more Jk^a antigen is present on the red cells of a Jk^aJk^a genotype individual than on the red cells of a Jk^aJk^b genotype person. The respective antibody therefore reacts stronger against the homozygote person's red cells compared with red cells from the heterozygote.

4. **List the antigens, which should be present on red cells used for antibody detection.**
C, c, D, E, e, K, k, Fy^a, Fy^b, Jk^a, Jk^b, S, s, M, N, P_1, Le^a and Le^b

5. **What antibody specificities are produced principally via pregnancy?**
Principally anti-D (and anti-C+D and anti-C+D+E). As Rh D negative blood is routinely transfused to D negative patients, anti-D is rarely stimulated as the result of a transfusion.

6. **Why is the antibody detection test potentially more important than the crossmatch for detecting alloantibodies?**
Red cell samples homozygous for selected antigen specificities are specially chosen for antibody detection and therefore they have maximal antigenic expression, i.e. D, c, Fy^a, Jk^a, Jk^b, S, s and Fy^b; whereas the donations selected for crossmatching may be heterozygous, and on a frequency basis are more likely to be so for certain specificities. A greater amount of antigen per red cell aids in antibody detection - especially for weak examples of certain antibodies which are susceptible to 'dosage effects' (e.g. anti-Kidd antibodies).

7. **What percentage of patients is likely to have a pre-formed alloantibody?**
Between 1-3% of all hospital patients have atypical antibodies in their serum/plasma.

8. **What does a positive crossmatch together with a negative antibody detection test result signify?**
- The wrong ABO group donation has been used for the crossmatch / wrongly labelled unit.
- A positive DAT donation

- That the patient has an alloantibody, the antigen to which is present on the blood unit selected for crossmatching but lacking from the antibody detection cell samples. This is likely to signify that the antibody in the patient's serum/plasma is reacting with a 'low-frequency' antigen present by chance on the donor's red cells. The specificity of the antibody should be identified and known antigen negative blood selected and crossmatched prior to transfusion.

9. **Outline the process by which antibodies are stimulated by pregnancy.**

Fetal red cells carrying paternally derived antigen(s) enter the maternal circulation during pregnancy due to a 'fetal bleed' and especially at delivery. These red cells 'survive normally' in the maternal circulation and may stimulate her to produce an alloantibody. This antibody may be stimulated by further pregnancies (all pregnancies will be antigen positive if the father is homozygous, 50% if he is heterozygous).

10. **Which blood donations are given additional (more sensitive) antibody screening tests?**

Donations intended for fetal / neonatal transfusion. This antibody screen is equivalent in sensitivity to that used for patients, to identify the presence of weak antibodies. The small recipient blood volume results in a possible increased chance of a minor transfusion reaction. (NOTE: these donations are also specific for additional criteria, e.g. irradiation, CMV negative, haemolysin poor, etc.).

ANTIBODY IDENTIFICATION

Patient Number 1

Antibodies identified:	Anti-D Anti-C indicated by a single positive reaction – ideally this needs confirming using a second D- C+ cell (r'r).
Antibodies masked:	Anti-C^w *
Antibodies excluded with only one positive example:	None
Antibodies excluded with only one homozygous example (i.e. S, s, Fy^a, Fy^b, Jk^a, Jk^b only):	None
Exclusions required (further red cells to be tested):	None (Kp^a *)
Blood selected for transfusion:	rr (CDE neg), ABO matched, crossmatch compatible (37°C, IAT).

Patient Number 2

Antibodies identified:	Anti-K
Antibodies masked:	Anti-Lu^a *
Antibodies excluded with only one positive example:	None
Antibodies excluded with only one homozygous example (i.e. S, s, Fy^a, Fy^b, Jk^a, Jk^b only):	None
Exclusions required (further red cells to be tested):	None (Kp^a *)
Blood selected for transfusion:	K-, ABO/D matched, crossmatch compatible (37°C, IAT).

Patient Number 3

Antibodies identified:	Anti-c
Antibodies masked:	Anti-E, anti-Lu^a *
Antibodies excluded with only one positive example:	N, P$_1$, K, Le^a, Le^b
Antibodies excluded with only one homozygous example (i.e. S, s, Fy^a, Fy^b, Jk^a, Jk^b only):	S, s, Fy^a, Fy^b, Jk^a, Jk^b
Exclusions required (further red cells to be tested):	As listed above, using a panel of c negative (R$_1$R$_1$) cells. The presence of anti-E can be determined using R$_1$R$_z$ or R$_z$R$_z$ cells (i.e. that are c-E+), however if c-E- blood is selected for the patient, this exclusion is not strictly necessary but should be done where possible. (Kp^a *)
Blood selected for transfusion:	c-E- ABO/D matched, crossmatch compatible (37°C, IAT). This is most likely to be R$_1$R$_1$ cells as a D-, c-person (Cde/Cde) would be very rare!

Patient Number 4

Antibodies identified:	Anti-Fy^a
Antibodies masked:	Anti-Lu^a *
Antibodies excluded with only one positive example:	K, Le^a, (D, E)
Antibodies excluded with only one homozygous example (i.e. S, s, Fy^a, Fy^b, Jk^a, Jk^b only):	s

Exclusions required (further red cells to be tested):	One Fy(a-) K+ cell One Fy(a-) Le(a+) cell One Fy(a-) S-s+ cell D and E : although only excluded with one cell by IAT the lack of reactivity in the enzyme panel excludes Rh antibody presence (this includes C^w). (Kp^a *)
Blood selected for transfusion:	Fy(a-), ABO/D matched, crossmatch compatible (37°C, IAT).

Patient Number 5

Antibodies identified:	Anti-M showing some 'dosage' (stronger reactions with M+N- (homozygous MM) cells, weaker reactions with M+N+ (heterozygous MN) cells).
Antibodies masked:	Anti-K, anti-Lu^a *
Antibodies excluded with only one positive example:	Le^a (D, C, E)
Antibodies excluded with only one homozygous example (i.e. S, s, Fy^a, Fy^b, Jk^a, Jk^b only):	Fy^a, Jk^a
Exclusions required (further red cells to be tested):	Two M- K+ cells One M- Le(a+) cell One M- Fy(a+b-) cell One M- Jk(a+b-) cell D, C and E : although only excluded with one cell by IAT the lack of reactivity in the enzyme panel excludes Rh antibody presence (this includes C^w). (Kp^a *)
Blood selected for transfusion:	M- ABO/D matched, crossmatch compatible (37°C, IAT).

Patient Number 6

Antibodies identified:	Anti-Jk^b showing some 'dosage' (stronger reactions with Jk(a-b+) cells, weaker reactions with Jk(a+b+) cells).
Antibodies masked:	Anti-Fy^a (if reacting with only homozygous Fy(a+b-) cells), anti-C^w *
Antibodies excluded with only one positive example:	C, N, Le^a
Antibodies excluded with only one homozygous example (i.e. S, s, Fy^a, Fy^b, Jk^a, Jk^b only):	S Anti-Fy^a is not excluded by any examples of homozygous Fy(a+b-) cells.
Exclusions required (further red cells to be tested):	Two Jk(b-), Fy(a+b-) cells One Jk(b-), C+ cell One Jk(b-), N+ cell One Jk(b-), Le(a+) cell One Jk(b-), S+s- cell (Kp^a *)
Blood selected for transfusion:	Jk(b-) ABO/D matched, crossmatch compatible (37°C, IAT).

Patient Number 7

Antibodies identified:	Anti-Le^b
Antibodies masked:	Anti-E, anti-s (if reacting with only homozygous ss (S-s+) cells)
Antibodies excluded with only one positive example:	D, C
Antibodies excluded with only one homozygous example (i.e. S, s, Fy^a, Fy^b, Jk^a, Jk^b only):	Fy^b, Jk^a Anti-s is not excluded by any examples of homozygous ss
Exclusions required (further red cells to be tested):	Two Le(b-) E+ cells Two Le(b-) S-s+ cells One Le(b-) D+ cell One Le(b-) C+ cell One Le(b-) Fy(a-b+) cell One Le(b-) Jk(a+b-) cell (Kp^a *)
Blood selected for transfusion:	ABO/D matched, crossmatch compatible (37°C, IAT). Note: Le(b-) is not required.

Patient Number 8

Antibodies identified:	Anti-e
Antibodies masked:	Anti-C, -C^w *, -M, -S, P$_1$, -Lu^a *, -K, -Le^a, -Jk^b. Anti-Fy^a or anti-Fy^b if reacting only with homozygous cells (i.e. Fy(a+b-) and Fy(a-b+) respectively).
Antibodies excluded with only one positive example:	D, E, c, N, Le^b
Antibodies excluded with only one homozygous example (i.e. S, s, Fy^a, Fy^b, Jk^a, Jk^b only):	s, Jk^a Anti-Fy^a or anti-Fy^b are not excluded by any examples of homozygous Fy(a+b-) or Fy(a-b+) cells respectively.
Exclusions required (further red cells to be tested):	Just about everything! In practice a panel of e- (R$_2$R$_2$) cells would be specifically selected to provide exclusions for the above listed specificities. (Kp^a *)
Blood selected for transfusion:	e- ABO/D matched, crossmatch compatible (37°C, IAT). This is most likely to be (R$_2$R$_2$) cells as a D-, e-person (cdE/cdE) would be very rare!

Patient Number 9

Antibodies identified:	Anti-S showing some 'dosage' (stronger reactions with S+s- (homozygous SS) cells, weaker reactions with S+s+ (heterozygous Ss) cells).
Antibodies masked:	Anti-Le^a, -Lu^a *
Antibodies excluded with only one positive example:	(C, E)
Antibodies excluded with only one homozygous example (i.e. S, s, Fy^a, Fy^b, Jk^a, Jk^b only):	Fy^b
Exclusions required (further red cells to be tested):	Two S- Le(a+) cells One S- Fy(a-b+) C and E : although only excluded with one cell by IAT the lack of reactivity in the enzyme panel excludes Rh antibody presence (this includes C^w). (Kp^a *)
Blood selected for transfusion:	S- ABO/D matched, crossmatch compatible (37°C, IAT).

Patient Number 10

Antibodies identified:	Anti-P$_1$
Antibodies masked:	Anti-K, anti--Lu^a *
Antibodies excluded with only one positive example:	C, Le^a
Antibodies excluded with only one homozygous example (i.e. S, s, Fy^a, Fy^b, Jk^a, Jk^b only):	Fy^b
Exclusions required (further red cells to be tested):	Two P$_1$- K+ cells One P$_1$- C+ cell One P$_1$- Le(a+) cell One P$_1$- Fy(a-b+) cell (Kp^a *)
Blood selected for transfusion:	ABO/D matched, crossmatch compatible (37°C, IAT). Note: P$_1$- is not required.

Patient Number 11

Antibodies identified:	Anti-D, anti-Fy^a and/or anti-s
Antibodies masked:	Anti-K, anti-C^w *, anti-Lu^a *
Antibodies excluded with only one positive example:	C, E, M, Le^a
Antibodies excluded with only one homozygous example (i.e. S, s, Fy^a, Fy^b, Jk^a, Jk^b only):	Jk^a
Exclusions required (further red cells to be tested):	To confirm the presence / absence of anti-Fy^a and/or anti-s there is a need to test against: Two D-, Fy(a-b+), S-s+ cells Two D-, Fy(a+b-), S+s- cells To exclude the other specificities, there is a need to test against the following: One D-, Fy(a-), s-, C+ cell One D-, Fy(a-), s-, E+ cell One D-, Fy(a-), s-, M+ cell One D-, Fy(a-), s- Le(a+) cell

	One D-, Fy(a-), s- Jk(a+b-) cell Note: if only anti-D+Fy^a is present, then the s-requirement is not necessary; if only anti-D+s is present, then the Fy(a-) requirement is not necessary. (Kp^a *)
Blood selected for transfusion:	D-, Fy(a-) and/or s- ABO/D matched, crossmatch compatible (37°C, IAT).

Patient Number 12

Antibodies identified:	Anti-Jk^a showing 'dosage' (i.e. only reacting with Jk(a+b-) cells and not at all with Jk(a+b+) cells)
Antibodies masked:	Anti-E, anti-Lu^a *
Antibodies excluded with only one positive example:	D
Antibodies excluded with only one homozygous example (i.e. S, s, Fy^a, Fy^b, Jk^a, Jk^b only):	None
Exclusions required (further red cells to be tested):	Two Jk(a-), E+ cells One Jk(a-), D+ cell (Kp^a *)
Blood selected for transfusion:	Jk(a-) ABO/D matched, crossmatch compatible (37°C, IAT).

Notes:
Due to the fact that antibodies have been detected in all of the above patients, in accordance with BCSH guideline for compatibility testing, a serological crossmatch is required (37°C IAT). This will also help to rule out the possible presence of any antibodies to low frequency antigens in the patient's plasma that have not been able to be identified by the antibody identification procedure. In other words if the blood selected happens to carry a low frequency antigen that corresponds with an antibody in the patient's plasma, then the crossmatch will be incompatible for that particular unit and therefore not transfused.

* Anti-Kp^a : this panel cannot rule out the presence of anti-Kp^a as well as antibodies to other low frequency antigen specificities that are not identified on the panel sheet (e.g. anti-Wr^a).
* Anti-C^w / anti-Lu^a : excluding the presence of these antibody specificities using specifically sub-grouped additional panel cells is not normally required due to their limited significance in transfusion and the fact that blood selected for transfusion will be serologically crossmatched.

Phenotyping the patient's red cells : it is recommended practice to antigen type the patient for the corresponding antibody found. This includes antithetical antigen typing. For example;
- If anti-Jk^a is detected the patient's red cells should be typed for Jk^a and Jk^b antigens.
- If anti-c is detected the patient's red cells should have a full Rh type performed, i.e. C, c, E, e antigen typing (note that D typing will already have been performed with the ABO group).
- If anti-S is detected the patient's cells should be typed for S and s antigens.

SECTION 8

1. **What pre-transfusion laboratory procedures are recommended?**
    - Checking the record of previous grouping and antibody screening results.
    - Performing ABO and D grouping.
    - Performing an antibody screening test.
    - Selection of blood and crossmatching the patient's serum/plasma against the donor's red cells, or using an 'electronic issue' system.

2. **What laboratory procedures should (in preference) be performed prior to an emergency transfusion?**
    ABO and D grouping the patient - issue ABO and RhD compatible units
    Antibody screen / IAT crossmatch pre blood issue (if possible).

3. **Explain the principles of the 'type and screen' procedure.**
    For many surgical procedures it is not necessary to have cross-matched blood immediately available for the patient. Therefore, in such cases, the patient's blood sample may be ABO/D grouped and antibody screened only. In such cases, should the patient subsequently need blood quickly, knowing their blood group and the fact that their antibody screen is negative means that blood can be provided by an immediate-spin crossmatch, an IAT crossmatch or electronic issue method, in the confident knowledge that the blood will be compatible.

4. **What is MSBOS and why is it used?**

Stands for 'maximum surgical blood order schedule' and is a scheme agreed with hospital medical staff, which lists the number of units of blood that should be routinely pre-operatively crossmatched for elective surgical procedures. The schedule is based on a retrospective analysis of actual blood used for different patient groups and in doing so attempts to match the amount of blood ordered with the amount actually used.

5. **How long should crossmatch work sheets be kept prior to disposal?**

The 'Guidelines on hospital blood bank documentation and procedures' (1990) identify that due to the Consumer Protection Act 'working documents should be retained for 11 years. The Report of the RCPath and IBMS (1999) 'The Retention of Pathological Records and Archives' (section C) states that worksheets and blood bank registers should be kept for 11 years, though results of grouping and antibody screening should be kept permanently. The Blood Safety and Quality Regulations (BSQR) 2005 (EC Commission Directive 2005/61/EC) states that hospitals should retain data for at least 30 years.

6. **What is an 'immediate spin' crossmatch and what is it primarily designed to detect?**

A saline test involving adding a volume of the patient's serum/plasma to a volume of suitably washed / diluted donor red cells, which are mixed and 'immediately' gently centrifuged. This test is used to detect possible ABO mismatches prior to transfusion - though its sensitivity, especially with respect to weak *in vitro* reactive antibodies, has been questioned.

7. **What is 'electronic issue'?**

This is where a patient with routine (confirmed) ABO and D group results and a negative antibody screening test has blood of the correct ABO/D group selected from the blood bank by a computer programme, without any serological crossmatching procedure having been performed. This is based on the understanding that any clinically important antibodies will be detected by the antibody detection procedure and that the majority of transfusion reaction incidents are due to ABO incompatibility, i.e. the computer programme ensures correct ABO/D group selection.

8. **Which blood group antibody specificities detected prior to crossmatch in a patient's serum/plasma requires the selection of antigen negative blood?**

Reactive at $37^{\circ}C$ by IAT. Guidelines for pre-transfusion testing indicates the following: Rh; Kell; Duffy; Kidd; S and s antibodies; anti-M reactive at $37^{\circ}C$ and antibodies against high / low frequency antigens (dependant upon specificity).

9. **Which antibody specificities are rarely 'clinically significant'?**

By comparison with question 8, those which are <u>not</u> reactive at $37^{\circ}C$ by IAT (though this is not always the case). This normally includes the following specificities: anti-A_1; -P_1; -N and some -M; -Le^a; -Le^b and -Le^{a+b}; HTLA and some antibodies against high / low frequency antigens (dependant upon specificity). In addition, anti-H/I (present in non-Bombay) and 'enzyme-only' antibodies (e.g. some anti-E).

10. **The visible inspection of blood donations prior to issue from the laboratory should ensure what?**

That there is no:
- Leakage from the ports or seams of the unit.
- Evidence of haemolysis in the plasma or at the interface between the red cells and plasma.
- Discolouration of the red cells.
- Presence of clots.

SECTION 9

1. **What is the major cause of severe immediate haemolytic transfusion reactions?**

Transfusion of ABO incompatible red cells, normally due to clerical error (related to incorrect patient identification).

2. **Explain the mechanism causing a delayed transfusion reaction to occur.**

Caused by a secondary immune response, when an antibody, previously present in the patient's serum/plasma is no longer detectable in pre-transfusion tests. As a result, antigen positive blood is transfused which re-stimulates antibody production. Following a delay, when enough antibody has been produced, the now incompatible red cells are destroyed, causing a fall in Hb and possible jaundice and fever.

3. **What is the most common error that results in a transfusion reaction?**

SHOT identifies that the most common error is that the incorrect blood component is transfused - this results from clerical error, either associated with patient identification, blood sample labelling and/or procedural errors involving the collection of blood from the hospital blood bank and its subsequent administration. A significant number of errors have been identified to have originated in the laboratory.

4. **TTI are reduced by what processes?**
   - Blood donor and donation screening procedures involving the pre-donation questioning / screening of the donor using the selection of donor guidelines and the exclusion of people within 'high-risk' groups.
   - All donations are mandatorily tested for the presence of the markers hepatitis B (HBV), hepatitis C (HCV), HIV, HTLV and syphilis (by EIA and NAT testing procedures).
   - The use of product viricidal treatment (e.g. methylene blue).

5. **What is TRALI and what causes it?**
   Transfusion related acute lung injury (TRALI) is an acute transfusion reaction characterised by the development of bilateral pulmonary infiltrates (nodules on the lung), which is associated with the reaction of a complement activating leucocyte specific antibody present in the plasma of the transfused component with the patient's WBCs. This 'minor' reaction results in the deposition of granulocytes in the patient's lung.

6. **What is PTP and what causes it?**
   Post-transfusion purpura (PTP) is thrombocytopenia occurring in a patient 5-12 days after a transfusion of a cellular product due to the reaction of a (pre-formed) platelet specific antibody in the patient reacting with transfused antigen positive platelets. The patient's own platelets may also be destroyed due to a 'bystander' reaction, producing the thrombocytopenia. The platelet antibody specificity is normally anti-HPA-1a, though other specificities may be involved.

7. **What is TA-GvHD and what causes it?**
   Transfusion-associated graft-versus-host-disease (TA-GvHD) is associated with the transfusion of viable WBCs, which produce an immune response against the recipient, which manifests itself by a variety of symptoms. The problem is removed by the irradiation of the product prior to transfusion, which inhibits DNA replication and therefore WBC cellular immune response (and GvHD) capability.

8. **Bacterial contamination of a blood donation can occur by what process?**
   - Contamination can occur from bacteria on the donor's skin, which is not removed by the cleaning technique used routinely prior to blood donation. These then enter the donation through the needle.
   - As a result of the donor having a symptom-free low-grade bacteraemia at the time of donation.
   - Contamination can also occur as a result of a blood bag manufacturing defect or processing defect involving the inadequately sealing of the bleed line - contamination entering the bag during storage.

9. **Identify the basic procedure for the investigation of a suspected immediate transfusion reaction.**
   Ensure that the following occurs:
   - The transfusion should be stopped and the nature of the adverse symptoms identified.
   - The unit being transfused (and giving set), together with the remains of the units of blood and/or blood products transfused prior to the reaction being identified, should be returned to the blood bank.
   - Fresh ('post-transfusion') blood sample should be taken from the patient.
   Basic procedure:
   - Check the patient's details against the units transfused and all other documentation to identify any clerical and/or labelling errors. If a clerical error is identified, ensure that checks are performed to exclude the involvement of another patient.
   - Centrifuge the post-transfusion sample and examine the serum/plasma for haemolysis.
   - Perform ABO and D grouping and a DAT on the patient's pre (laboratory stored) and post-transfusion blood samples and each of the transfused units, including those units transfused prior to the one suspected of causing the reaction.
   - Repeat the antibody screening tests on both the pre and post-transfusion patient serum/plasma samples and repeat crossmatch all units with both the pre and post-transfusion samples.
   - If appropriate, check the blood units transfused for bacterial contamination.
   - In the absence of red cell incompatibility - tests to identify the presence of WBC and/or platelet antibodies in the patient's pre-transfusion blood sample.
   If any evidence is identified to suggest that an error has occurred, report to senior scientific and medical staff who will decide on any appropriate action, including implementation of changes as necessary to procedures and report the incident to the SHOT scheme.

10. **Why is a positive DAT result 'mixed field' in a delayed transfusion reaction?**
As additional antibody is produced in response to the transfusion, it binds with the antigen positive transfused red cells. It is these red cells, which when coated with sufficient amounts of antibody, react positively in the DAT. This combination of negative patient cells and positive reacting transfused cells results in the 'mixed field' effect. The ratio of positive to negative red cells (and therefore the degree of the mixed field effect) will vary dependant upon the patient's blood volume and the amount transfused. It also varies within each patient with time as the antibody is initially produced and binds in increasing quantities to the transfused red cells and is recognised by the DAT, and then subsequently as the red cells are removed from the patient's circulation.

SECTION 10

1. **List the 'major blood group systems' and their principal antigens.**

SYSTEM NAME	MAJOR ANTIGENS
ABO	A, B
Rh	C, c, D, E, e
MNS	M, N, S, s
P	P_1
Kell	K, k, Js^a, Js^b, Kp^a, Kp^b
Duffy	Fy^a, Fy^b
Kidd	Jk^a, Jk^b
Lewis	Le^a, Le^b
Lutheran	Lu^a, Lu^b

2. **List the antigens that are destroyed by proteolytic enzymes, such as papain.**
M, N, S, (s), Fy^a, Fy^b

3. **Why is anti-k such a rare antibody?**
Only 0.2% of the population have the genotype *KK* and these are the only people able to produce anti-k when immunised. In addition, the k antigen is a poor immunogen.

4. **Why is anti-K such a common antibody?**
The K antigen is a strong immunogen (only A/B and Rh antigens are stronger) and as such readily stimulates antibody; in addition approximately 9 out of 10 people are K-negative and therefore a large number of people are capable of producing the antibody.

5. **What blood group donations should be selected for a group A Rh D positive patient with anti-Fy^a reactive by AHG at 37°C and anti-A_1 reactive by saline techniques at 20°C?**
Group A Rh D positive Fy(a-b+) blood is required since the anti-Fy^a is clinically important and antigen negative blood is required. The anti-A_1 is not clinically important and crossmatch compatible blood is sufficient to ensure that the red cells will survive normally in the patient.

6. **How does an antibody to a high frequency antigen normally react in pre-transfusion tests. How is its specificity identified?**
The ABO and D groups normally give expected normal reactions if the antibody is reactive at 37°C. The antibody detection test is positive by AHG technique vs. all cell samples used. On using a cell identification panel, all red cell samples are also normally positive (as are all donations used for crossmatching), however the DAT / auto controls are negative indicating the antibody to be non-auto. Elucidation of the antibody specificity requires the use of a specially selected cell panel, which is chosen to contain red cells that lack high frequency antigens (referral to a reference laboratory is required). The method is employed in an attempt to identify a red cell sample, which gives a negative result. The patient's red cells can also be grouped for high frequency antigens to identify any negative result. Anti-H / anti-I may be detected by additional reactions of cells used in the serum ABO group. Anti-H antibodies may be identified by their weaker reaction with group A_1 red cells and anti-I by its negative (weaker) result with group O cord red cells.

7. **Which of the major blood group system antibodies are not normally clinically significant?**
Anti-A_1; anti-P_1 and anti-Le^b and cold reactive anti-H/I are not normally clinically significant.
Anti-N and anti-M if un-reactive at 37°C are not clinically significant.
Anti-Le^a and anti-Le^{a+b} are rarely clinically significant.
HTLA antibodies are unlikely to be clinically important.
(see also Section 7: Pre-transfusion testing).

8. **Which is the most common Duffy genotype in White and Black populations?**
The most common group in Whites is Fy(a+b+) (genotype Fy^aFy^b) at approximately 47% and the rarest is Fy(a-b-) (genotype $FyFy$) at <0.1%. Conversely, the most common group in Blacks is Fy(a-b-) at approximately 76% in some Black populations in West Africa, whereas the rarest is Fy(a+b+) at approximately 1%. This reversal in phenotype frequencies is believed to be associated with the fact that Fy(a-b-) red cells are resistant to invasion by the malarial parasites *Plasmodium knowlesi* (*in vitro*) and *Plasmodium vivax* (*in vivo*), i.e. it is advantageous for Black Africans to lack Duffy red cell antigens.

9. **Which of the following antibodies are classified as 'clinically significant'?**

a.	Anti-Jk^a	Yes
b.	Anti-Fy^b	Yes
c.	Anti-M (reactive at 37°C)	Yes
d.	Anti-Lu^b	Variably (seek advice from Transfusion Centre)

10. **Why is it possible for a RBC Lewis group to change from Le(a-b+) to Le(a-b-)?**
Due to the fact that the antigens are adsorbed onto the red cells from the plasma in variable amounts. This may result (under certain circumstances) in the red cell Lewis phenotype of a person becoming weaker or even 'disappearing'. This is most frequently seen in pregnancy and in patients on steroid therapy.

SECTION 11

1. **What antibody specificity causes the most serious / major HDFN? Why is this?**
Anti-D (anti-C+D etc.). High immunogenicity results in antibody production if the mother is D negative and the fetal cells D positive; antibody is frequently IgG and therefore able to cross the placenta. The D antigen is well expressed in early fetal life. The antibody is capable of destroying fetal red cells.

2. **Which blood group system is the most frequent cause of HDFN? Why is this?**
ABO. ABO incompatibility between mother and fetus is common (e.g. group O mother and group A baby) and this can give rise to mild HDFN due to maternal IgG anti-A,B crossing the placenta and binding to fetal red cells. Mild effects due to neutralisation of maternal antibody by non-red cell antigen, low amount of maternal IgG ABO antibody in many women and poor development of fetal A/B red cell antigens are factors.

3. **What levels of anti-D is associated with:**

• Low risk of HDFN?	Less than 4 IU/mL
• Mild to moderate risk of HDFN?	4 –15 IU/mL
• High risk of HDFN?	Above 15 IU/mL

4. **When should anti-D immunoglobulin be given?**
Antenatally: routinely when the mother is D negative (with no pre-formed anti-D antibody) as two doses at 28 and 34 weeks or one larger dose at 28 weeks and non-routinely to D negative women (with no pre-formed anti-D antibody) within 72 hours of a 'potentially sensitising episode' (does based on Kleihauer).
Post-natally: within 72 hours of delivery to D negative woman (with no pre-formed anti-D antibody) who has given birth to a D positive baby (dose based on Kleihauer)

5. **What test is performed to identify the amount of a feto-maternal bleed?**
A Kleihauer-Betke test or the use of a Flow Cytometer.

6. **Feto-maternal haemorrhage most commonly occurs at delivery. What other conditions can lead to a feto-maternal haemorrhage?**
Potential feto-maternal sensitising episodes occurring during pregnancy:
   • Therapeutic termination of pregnancy
   • Ectopic pregnancy
   • Spontaneous (complete or incomplete) abortion (>12 weeks)
   • Amniocentesis
   • Chorionic villus sampling
   • Fetal blood sampling
   • Intrauterine bleeding (>12 weeks) / antepartum haemorrhage
   • External cephalic version of the fetus
   • Closed abdominal surgery
   • Intrauterine death
   • Miscarriage / stillbirth
   • Manual removal of placenta
   • Abdominal trauma

7. **Should anti-D prophylaxis be offered to an Rh D negative mother with anti-D who has delivered an Rh D positive baby? Explain the reasons for your answer.**

No. The mother has already produced the antibody and her immune response has been stimulated, therefore the Ig will be ineffective.

8. **Following the detection of a 37°C IAT reactive antibody in an antenatal blood sample, what further action should be taken?**

Organise additional blood samples at regular intervals – every 4 weeks during the first two trimesters of pregnancy and from 28 weeks, every 2 weeks. Confirm the antibody specificity and quantify (as IU/mL if anti-D or anti-c) or perform a titration for non-Rh antibodies. Dependant upon the antibody specificity detected, test the father for his red cell genotype.

9. **What options are available to treat severe HDFN?**

Dependant upon the degree of anaemia:
- Intrauterine transfusion, IUT, to prevent the fetus becoming too anaemic.
- Immediate exchange transfusion after delivery, to treat anaemia.
- Exchange transfusion to prevent the bilirubin becoming too high (by removing the plasma containing bilirubin and the sensitised red cells that are 'potential' bilirubin.
- Possible simple, top-up, transfusions several days post delivery to correct anaemia.

10. **How does anti-K cause HDFN?**

It binds to red cell precursors in the bone marrow and suppresses red cell production, which leads to anaemia.

SECTION 12

1. **What are the 4 main reasons for *in vivo* mediated red cell destruction?**
   - Transfused red cells being destroyed by an antibody the individual has produced (HTR)
   - Fetal red cells being destroyed by a maternal antibody (HDFN)
   - An individuals red cells being destroyed by an auto-antibody they have produced – autoimmune haemolytic anaemia (AIHA)
   - An individual's red cells being destroyed by an antibody derived from donor lymphocytes in a transplant or transplanted donor. Red cells being destroyed by an antibody from the recipient.

2. **What is the direct antiglobulin test used for and what are its limitations?**

The direct antiglobulin test (DAT) is used to test red cells directly, without any *in vitro* incubation, to detect antibodies and /or complement that has been bound *in vivo*. The DAT is used in the investigation of cases of suspected immune red cell destruction. However a positive DAT, in itself, is not diagnostic of a *haemolytic anaemia*, as there also has to be evidence of increased red cell destruction, such as a low Hb, raised reticulocyte count, reduced haptoglobins, raised bilirubin, and raised LDH. A DAT should be performed using a polyspecific AHG reagent that contains both anti-IgG and anti-C3, as these are often found on red cells from patients with immune red cell destruction. The DAT can also be performed with monospecific reagents that include at least anti-IgG and anti-C3 but might include anti-IgA and anti-IgM.

3. **What are the main characteristics of warm AIHA?**

This is the most common type of AIHA and is caused by an IgG autoantibody; sometimes C3 is also present. The DAT is positive with anti-IgG and possibly anti-C3. Red cells coated with IgG are removed in the spleen but if complement coated, there might be more rapid cell destruction in the liver. In some cases IgM or IgA antibodies may be found in addition to IgG and very rarely IgA might be present on its own, detected by using a monospecific anti-IgA reagent. The autoantibodies found in warm AIHA often have a Rh-related specificity e.g. auto-anti-e or 'e-like'. Although some cases of warm AIHA are *idiopathic*, occurring without any obvious underlying cause, most cases of positive DATs now seen are related to haematological malignancies, e.g. MDS.

4. **What are the main characteristics of cold AIHA?**

In cold AIHA antibodies are not usually detected on the cells by the DAT but C3 is present indicating that an antigen-antibody reaction has taken place by a cold-reacting IgM autoantibody, often anti-I or anti-i. These antibodies react with the patient's own cells in the peripheral capillaries, such as the finger tips, where the blood might be at 30°C rather than 37°C. This initiates the complement cascade and as the blood returns to the warmer parts of the body the antibody elutes from the cells but as the complement cascade has been started it might, in extreme cases, go to completion resulting in *intravascular* lysis or rapid lysis in the liver. When this happens the patient can present with haemoglobinuria after exposure to the cold. In less extreme cases the complement cascade is halted at the C3 stage and C3d is found on the red cells that probably have a near normal half-life.

5. **What are the main characteristics of PCH?**
PCH is caused by a bi-phasic, IgG antibody, usually anti-P; the so called Donath-Landsteiner antibody. The antibody reacts in the cold and activates complement in the warm leading to haemolysis and haemoglobinuria. The diagnostic test is the D-L test. Although classically associated with syphilis this condition is now almost always seen in children and often associated with a viral infection. Although it is self-limiting, that is resolves after a few days, some patients do present with acute haemolysis that requires transfusion.

6. **What are the main characteristics of drug induced / associated haemolytic anaemia?**
   - Drug-dependent type:
     Antibodies react mainly against the drug coating the red cells; e.g. the penicillins and cephalosporins. The DAT is usually positive with IgG, sometimes C3. Haemolysis develops slowly but can be life threatening.
   - Immune complex mechanism:
     Drug immune complexes attach to the cell surface can result in acute haemolysis with haemoglobinuria and renal failure. Severe haemolytic episodes can recur even with small doses of the drug. The DAT is usually positive with C3, but with some drugs, IgM or IgG can be detected. The antibody only reacts with drug-coated cells.
   - Drug independent antibodies:
     The drug stimulates an antibody that reacts with the red cell membrane not the drug itself. This type can not be distinguish from warm AIHA as the cells react with anti-IgG. The serum and eluate also react with normal red cells without the drug having to be present. This type was more common when methyldopa was widely used as a drug.
   - Non-immunological protein adsorption:
     Some cephalosporins can alter the cell membrane causing non-specific uptake of proteins including IgG and IgM, which are detectable by the DAT.

7. **Is the DAT always positive in cases of AIHA?**
No, there are cases where a patient has clinical AIHA but the DAT using a polyspecific AHG is negative. Some of these have been shown, on further investigation, to have IgA on the cell surface, but in others it is assumed that either low-affinity autoantibodies are involved or there are low levels of IgG1 or 3 that are not detectable in the standard DAT.

8. **If the DAT is positive is there always increased red cell destruction?**
No, there are cases where the DAT is positive but there is no increased red cell destruction. For example, with the use of the therapeutic immunoglobulin preparations (anti-lymphocyte and anti-thymocyte globulins), the immunoglobulins 'stick' to the red cells in a non-specific manner. Also a number of patients and donors have a positive DAT with no evidence of increased cell destruction. The reason might be that the cells are coated with IgG4 molecules that seem not to initiate cell destruction.

9. **Why can immune haemolysis occur after a transplant?**
In minor mismatches the donor can produce antibodies to the recipient's red cells, as in an O donor / A recipient. This is usually noticed between 5-15 days post transplant, with a rapidly falling Hb and possible renal failure. Anti-A or anti-B produced by lymphocytes transfused with the bone marrow, so called 'passenger lymphocytes'. The haemolysis subsides as the patient's remaining incompatible red cells are destroyed and replaced with those of donor origin. During the haemolytic episode the DAT may be positive and the causative antibody eluted from the patient's red cells.

In major mismatches the recipient can produce antibodies to the donor cells, as in an A donor and O recipient, where the donor's red cells are destroyed by the recipient's ABO antibodies. This might lead to the delay in the production of the donor red cells or as erythropoesis increases the residual antibodies might lyse these cells; haemolysis is not noted until 30-100 weeks after the transplant. The DAT is usually positive with IgG anti-A/B being eluted. In both minor and major mis-matches ABO antibodies are most common but other antibodies, Rh, Kidd, Lewis, have been reported.

Autoimmune haemolytic anaemia post transplant is rare; the donor's immune cells produce antibodies directed at the donor red cells; usually 10 or so months post BMT.

10. **Why are alloantibodies more important than autoantibodies when crossmatching blood for a patient with AIHA?**
In AIHA the patient's own red cells are being destroyed by the autoantibody and transfused cells would be destroyed at the same rate. If there was an alloantibody also present this could destroy any incompatible transfused cells at an increased rate and possibly exacerbate the AIHA. Transfusions should be avoided and other treatments used but if blood is needed the presence of alloantibodies, which may be masked by unbound autoantibody, have to be excluded by using absorption techniques. If an alloantibody is detected then antigen negative blood should be used.

SECTION 13

1. **List the mandatory tests carried out on all donations.**
   - ABO and Rh D group by sensitive methods.
   - Atypical red cell antibody screen.
   - Microbiology (Virology) tests : EIA / NAT
     - HBsAg (hepatitis B antigen).
     - HCV and anti-HCV (hepatitis C and antibody to hepatitis C).
     - Anti-HIV 1 and 2 (antibody to HIV).
     - HTLV
     - A test for syphilis antibody (i.e. TpHA or similar).

2. **What procedures may be employed for reducing the possibility of disease transmission by transfusion?**
   - Improving donor selection
   - Improving donation testing
   - Quarantining of donations
   - Reducing inappropriate transfusions
   - Autologous transfusion where appropriate
   - Product processing
   - Viral inactivation processing of products

3. **What steps are taken to minimise the possible bacterial contamination of platelets?**
   - Improved skin cleansing of donor's arm / venepuncture site
   - Pre-donation donor health check questionnaire - identification of people attending to give blood who may have bacteria in their bloodstream
   - Contaminated collection equipment / contamination during component processing - the sterilisation of collection packs by manufacturers fails or processing causes failure in seals
   - Diversion of the first few millilitres of blood away from the donation pack into the test sample tubes
   - Testing for the presence of bacteria in the final product
   - Pathogen inactivation by the treatment of the product
   - Pre-issue visual check by Blood Centre / Blood Bank staff

4. **Why must blood products for neonatal use have an extra red cell antibody test?**
   The standard antibody test performed on donations uses an enzyme system optimised to detect Rh and K antibodies. It will not detect weak antibodies or antibodies requiring an IAT for their detection. The expectation is that these antibodies, if present, will be diluted sufficiently in an adult's circulation to not cause clinical symptoms. For neonates, the dilution effect is absent because of their small size. It is important to use an antibody test that can detect these antibodies (e.g. anti-Fy^a, anti-S) using a sensitive antiglobulin based test, with un-pooled reagent cells having homozygous expression of all common Rh and other antigens (K may be heterozygote), so as to detect those antibodies that are active at 37^oC and are potentially clinically significant.

5. **Why is it important to detect donors who are DVI? What Rh type should the blood pack from such a donor be labelled as?**
   DVI is the commonest of the partial D types. People with variant D lack one or more components (epitopes) of the D antigen. The remaining part is still potentially immunogenic, so if transfused to a D negative patient can stimulate production of anti-D, which may cause HDFN or a transfusion reaction. It is therefore important to detect partial D, especially DVI and label the products from such donors as RhD positive.

6. **What is the current sensitivity required for HBsAg screening assays used to test donors? How do we prove this level of sensitivity is achieved?**
   Current 'Red Book' requirements for HBsAg assays used for testing donations have a sensitivity of at least 0.2 IU/mL for HBsAg. An independent 0.21 IU/mL standard is available from NIBSC and must be included in each batch of tests. For the tests to be considered valid the standard must be positive. For ELISA tests, a batch is defined as every plate or part plate. For Prism™, a batch is defined as all tests run with one set of calibrators.

7. **A hospital transfusion laboratory contacts you about a patient with anti-Kp^a in their serum and asks for typed red cells to be provided. What answer would you give the laboratory and why?**
   Kp^a is an antigen of the Kell blood group system. Antibodies to Kp^a are active at 37^oC and have been associated with both HDFN and HTR. However, the frequency of the antigen in the UK population is only ~2%. Advice to the hospital laboratory would be that screened (antigen negative) units would not be provided as crossmatching banked blood would be expected to provide suitable units for transfusion.

8. **Give two reasons why HbS screening of red cells may be performed.**
   HbS screening may be performed:
   - On red cell products for neonatal use.
   - On red cell products for patients with sickle cell disease or thalassaemia.
   - On donations from ethnic groups (with their permission). Positives have a higher risk of leuco-reduction filter failure, so all products from HbAS donors have a post-filtration white cell count performed on them.

9. **Briefly describe how Statistical Process Monitoring aids quality in the performance of microbiology immuno-assays.**
   Statistical Process Monitoring (SPM) is a 'trending tool' to look for performance variation over time. By plotting the sample / cut-off ratio for each NIBSC working standard in a spreadsheet (using a piece of software like Quality Analyst) the system can be set to allow calculation of a mean line as well as upper and lower control limits. By looking for non-random activity it is possible to pre-empt a possible system failure. Non-random conditions prompt an investigation into the cause, which may identify that equipment needs servicing or repair before degradation becomes critical. The fact that a batch of tests is 'out-of-control' does not mean that the batch has failed, providing that manufacturer's control and quality requirements are met and the working standard is positive.

10. **What is the 'window period' of a transfusion transmitted infection?**
    The time between infection of a person and the first detectable marker of disease. A donation given in this period may be infective as the microbiology test result will be negative.

11. **Why is NAT testing done for hepatitis C but not for hepatitis B?**
    The driving force for introducing NAT testing is the European Pharmacopoeia which requires start pools for manufacturing medicinal products to be tested for HCV RNA by a validated method. The initial instruction from the European Committee on Proprietary Medicines (ECPM) followed a number of outbreaks of HCV infection in recipients of blood products, which had been made from anti-HCV negative donations. As sensitive tests were already in place for HBV this reason to test by NAT did not arise for this agent.

12. **List the steps involved in the PCR test used for hepatitis C testing of blood donations and give a brief explanation of each.**
    There are four basic steps to the method:
    a. Extraction:
       This step is used to extract and concentrate nucleic acid from sample. It will extract all nucleic acids present, both DNA and RNA.
    b. Reverse transcription:
       As PCR only amplifies DNA, when looking for RNA viruses such as HCV and HIV, this step is required to make a DNA copy of the RNA using the enzyme reverse transcriptase. This type of assay is called rtPCR. When looking for DNA viruses such as HBV this step is not required.
    c. Amplification:
       The extracted DNA is heated to separate the two strands then cooled. A replicating enzyme such as taq polymerase is added along with a supply of bases and primer sequences specific to the virus(es) under investigation. This causes a copy of the two DNA strands to be made, doubling the concentration.
    d. Detection:
       A specific viral DNA sequence is tagged with a marker and used as a probe. This probe binds to the amplified viral DNA, if present, and allows detection of the reaction. For blood screening, the favoured probe is HRP, which is used to produce a colour reaction just like in EIA tests.

13. **Why might leucodepletion improve the microbiological safety of blood donations?**
    Certain viruses (and bacteria) are found in the white cells and are removed along with them during leucodepletion, e.g. CMV, HTLV-1, a proportion of HIV, etc.

14. **What is the current estimated risks of a patient contracting hepatitis B, HIV and hepatitis C respectively from a unit of blood in the UK?**
    Hepatitis B: 1 in 500,000
    HIV: 1 in 5,220,000
    Hepatitis C: 1 in 29,030,000

SECTION 14

1. **List the storage criteria for 'red cells for transfusion'.**
   Storage cabinets for red cells should comply with the British Standard BS4376 (part 1). The air temperature must be maintained between 2°C and 8°C (storage temperature 4°C $\pm$ 2°C) and an alarm

must sound if the temperature goes outside this range. A thermograph should record the temperature of a simulated product (a temperature probe in 100 ml of water).

2. **What are the advantages of producing SAG-M red cells?**
   - More plasma can be removed from each whole blood donation for fractionation.
   - Adenine is added to red cells after plasma removal.
   - SAG-M suspended red cells have a flow rate approaching that expected of whole blood.

3. **Identify the factors that affect the pH of stored platelet concentrates.**
   Anticoagulant: buffering effects
   Mixing: reduces the amount of anaerobic respiration
   Volume/concentration: optimal platelet number to plasma volume ratio
   Plastic pack: gas permeability

4. **Identify the additional criteria required of products intended for neonatal use.**
   Requirements for products used for IUT and exchange transfusions:
   As well as requiring the mandatory donation testing and product preparation procedures, also require all of the following:
   - Prepared from a donation provided by a donor who has given a previous donation
   - Leucodepleted ($<5 \times 10^6$ leucocytes)
   - Tested and found to be CMV antibody negative
   - Identified to be free of clinically significant red cell alloantibodies (as tested by sensitive antibody detection technique(s), equivalent to those used for the pre-transfusion testing of patients)
   - HbS negative (where indicated)
   - Identified to be free of high titre 'haemolysin' ABO antibodies
   - All cellular products to be gamma-irradiated prior to transfusion and used within 24 hours of irradiation.
   - To be prepared as a smaller volume in a concentrated form (e.g. RBCs should be plasma depleted).
   - Red cells to be less than 5 days old at the time of transfusion and free of additive solution (SAG-M)
   Products used for top-up transfusions:
   Products used for this purpose do not require the same criteria and the following are the differences from the requirements for products used for IUT/exchange transfusion:
   - No need for absence of high titre anti-A / anti-B
   - Red cells in additive solution (SAG-M) may be used
   - Product does not require gamma-irradiation (unless an exchange transfusion has been given at an earlier time)
   - Red cells up to 35 days expiry may be used

5. **What are 'specific human immunoglobulins' and what are they used for?**
   Fractionated plasma product produced from pooled plasma which are known to contain specific high titre antibodies, produced as a result of previous infection or active immunisation. Produced to provide passive immunisation against a variety of infections, e.g. rabies. Rh immunoglobulin is prepared from selected pooled plasma donations known to contain anti-D and increasing from manufactures monoclonal antibody preparations, is used for the prevention of HDFN.

6. **Complete a table of product storage criteria:**

	Temperature	Lifetime
Red cells:	$4^{\circ}C \pm 2^{\circ}C$	35 days
Platelets:	$22^{\circ}C \pm 2^{\circ}C$	5 days
FFP:	below $-30^{\circ}C$	2 years
Cryoprecipitate:	below $-30^{\circ}C$	2 years
HAS:	$20^{\circ}C$	3 years

7. **Reconstituted frozen red cells are used for transfusion to what type of patient?**
   Used for the storage of rare red cell phenotypes and therefore transfused to patients with an antibody to a high frequency antigen and also for patients with multiple antibody specificities. Also for autologous transfusion.

8. **What are the principle constituents of cryoprecipitate?**
   Factor VIII and fibrinogen.

9. **What are the three main categories of protein concentrate produced by fractionation of plasma?**
   Coagulation factors, immunoglobulins and albumin HAS.

10. **What is the minimum number of granulocytes in a granulocyte concentrate and how are these produced?**
To contain as a minimum 5×10^9 per unit; by pooling of donations or apheresis.

SECTION 15

1. **Define the terms quality assurance and quality control.**
Quality Assurance:
All those planned and systematic actions necessary to provide adequate confidence that a product or service will satisfy given requirements for quality.
Quality Control:
The operational techniques and activities that are used to fulfil requirements for quality.

2. **What are the differences between internal and external quality schemes?**
External quality assessment (EQA) refers to a system of retrospectively and objectively comparing results obtained from different laboratories by means of exercises organised by an external agency (UK NEQAS). Internal quality control refers to a prospective system designed to indicate the acceptability of a particular result, related to the performance of reagents, techniques, equipment and people.

3. **In what ways are the hospital blood banks "keepers" of blood and blood products?**
Under 'Product Liability' laws, each person or organisation in the chain of supply has a responsibility as a 'keeper' of a product, even if they are not the actual producer. Therefore, the hospital blood bank has a 'duty of care' to ensure that the blood/blood products that it keeps are suitable for their intended use. To do this the blood bank needs to maintain accurate records of what it receives and when (i.e. date and time), how these products are stored and how/when they are used/disposed of or returned to the supplier.

4. **What is CPA and what does it do?**
Clinical Pathology Accreditation (UK) Ltd is a voluntary peer review audit system against a series of guidelines / standards used for pathology departments.

5. **What is MHRA and what does it do?**
Good Manufacturing Practice (Rules and Guidance for Pharmaceutical Manufacturers and Distributors), is written by the Medicines & Healthcare products Regulatory Agency (MHRA). Blood Centres must be licensed under the Medicines Act – are audited every two years (minimum) by the MCA to ensure compliance (mandatory). The GMP guide includes sections on quality management, personnel, premises and equipment, documentation and production. Hospital Blood Banks are subject to audit by the MHRA as a result of the introduction of BSQR (2005).

6. **Why are SOPs important? What are the possible consequences of not following a particular SOP?**
An SOP is an instructional document, written to ensure a user can perform a task according to requirements. All SOPs must be validated to ensure the required outcome is achieved. These are given a unique number and are subject to regular review. It is the responsibility of all persons to ensure that SOPs are followed correctly and are not subject to unauthorised alterations. The consequences of not following a particular SOP are a lack of consistency, change in sensitivity and possible error.

7. **Identify what documents control a 'Quality System'.**
Two main documents:
The Quality Manual – a managerial statement of intent, available to all staff which defines:
- Management responsibilities
- Control of purchasing
- Documentation of procedures
- Equipment maintenance / calibration
- Product monitoring, handling, storage and traceability
- Records maintenance
- Staff training
The Document Control Policy: this is a policy defining how documents (e.g. SOPs, Forms, etc.) within the department are:
- Uniquely identified (i.e. number and version)
- Written (e.g. in what format)
- Validated
- Approved
- Issued
- Reviewed (e.g. annually)

8. **Identify the essential aspects of a Standard Operating Procedure (SOP) document.**

   A Standard Operating Procedure (SOP) is an instructional document, written to ensure a user can perform a task according to requirements. The author should be familiar with both the procedure and the required format (in which the SOP should be written). All SOPs must be validated (i.e. the procedure is performed by a second party who follows the instructions as laid out in the document) to ensure the required outcome is achieved. In addition, the SOP must be approved by a responsible manager to ensure that the requirements of the department are being met in the document. SOPs must be given a unique number; copies issued to named persons and be subject to regular review. It is also the responsibility of all persons to ensure that SOPs are followed correctly and are not subjected to unauthorised alterations.

9. **Define Good Manufacturing Practice (GMP).**

   That part of quality assurance, which ensures that products are consistently produced and controlled to the quality standards appropriate to their intended use. (The GMP Guide, Rules and Guidance for Pharmaceutical Manufacturers, contains a section on the manufacture of blood products).

10. **Why are clear and accurate records important?**
    - Enables people to be clear about what they, and other people, are doing.
    - Confirms what has been done, and by whom.
    - Important in the investigation of any complaints, defects, problems, etc.
    - Helps people take necessary corrective action.

213